JOAN OLIPHANT-[illegible] vintage, one, which has been said, combined [illegible] iquet of 1884 with the body and richness of 1893.

She received a diploma in Oenology in Paris and many magnums later became a Member Judge of the Club Oenologique in England, and is a contributor to the recently published Wheeler's Anthology, Oysters and Champagne.

Her other love is movement which embraces all sorts of dancing and in more recent years, as a result of gourmet activities, various types of exercise to keep slender, youthful and supple.

A great believer in deep breathing she is an advocate of fresh air and the outdoor life and can think of nothing better than a simple little meal prepared by a great Chef accompanied by a couple of bottles of de Luxe Champagne lovingly consumed half way up (or down) a mountain.

Described as a Slender Gourmet she would like to spread the word that you can indulge and shed the pounds at the same time.

MICHAEL FFOLKES was born in London in 1925, a short distance from the grape as the crow flies.

Long convinced of the delights of Champagne he was unaware of its dietetic virtues until the Authoress brought them to his attention. This has naturally redoubled his enthusiasm for the frequent glass or two.

To keep slimmer he indulges in mad solo dancing to any lively music (preferably New Orleans jazz) that comes on the radio and feels this may complement the exercises described within.

My life has been a love affair with champagne
and I would like to dedicate this book
to my favourite eight 'grandes marques'

Laurent-Perrier
Roederer
G. H. Mumm
Heidsieck
Tattinger
Piper Heidsieck
Henriot
Perrier Jouet

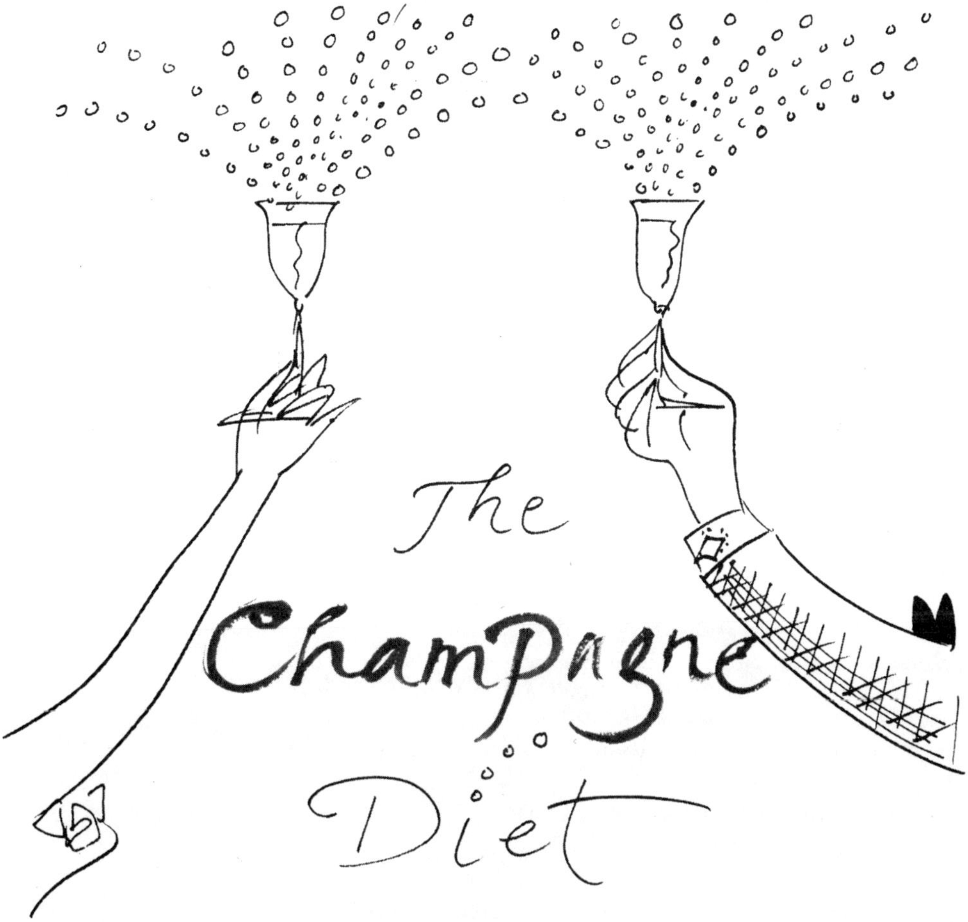

The Champagne Diet

by

The Slender Gourmet

JOAN OLIPHANT-FRASER

DEBRETT'S PEERAGE LIMITED
LONDON • NEW YORK • SYDNEY • PERTH W.A.

ISBN 0 905649 89 3
Published by Debrett's Peerage Limited,
73 – 77 Britannia Road, London SW6 2JR

Represented by Michael Joseph Limited,
27 Wright's Lane, Kensington, London W8

Distributed by TBL Book Distribution Services,
17 – 23 Nelson Way, Tuscan Trading Estate, Camberley, Surrey

Designed by Andrew Ivett
Typeset in Sabon by Holywell Press Ltd, Oxford
Printed and bound in Great Britain by R. J. Acford, Chichester, Sussex

'O! that this too solid flesh would melt . . .'
Hamlet, Act I, Scene II

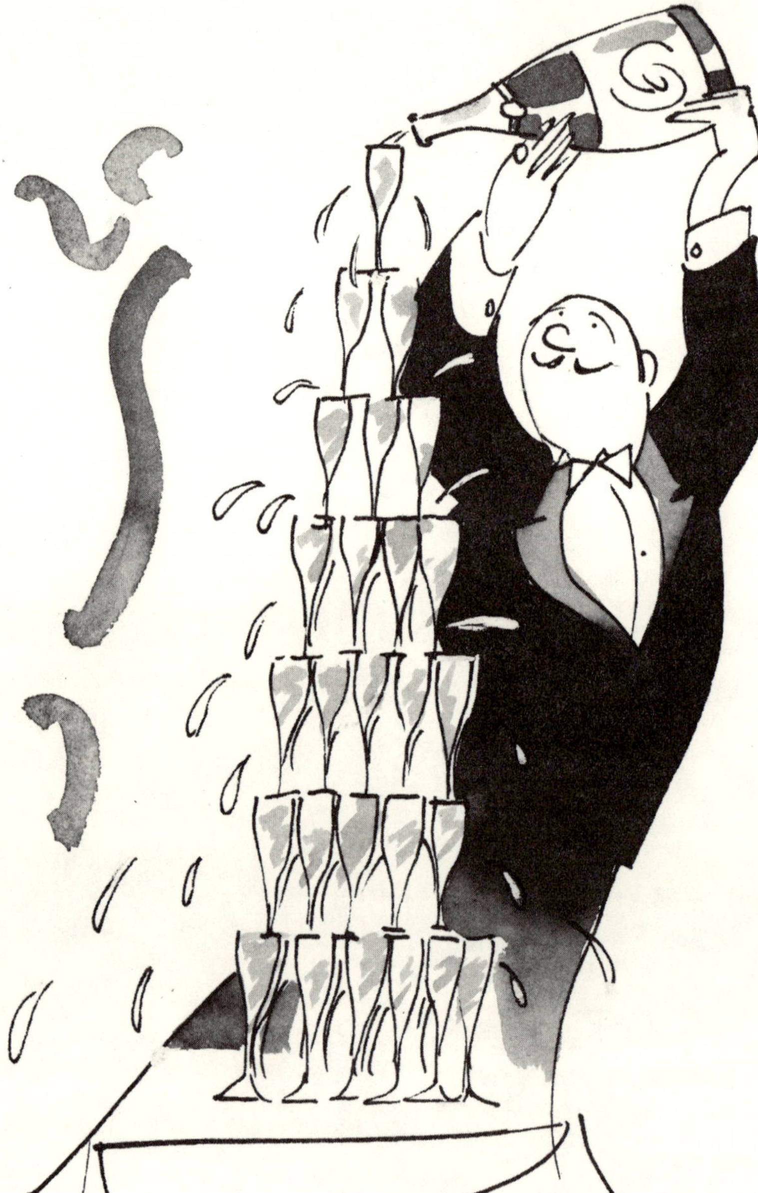

Fontaine de Champagne

Contents

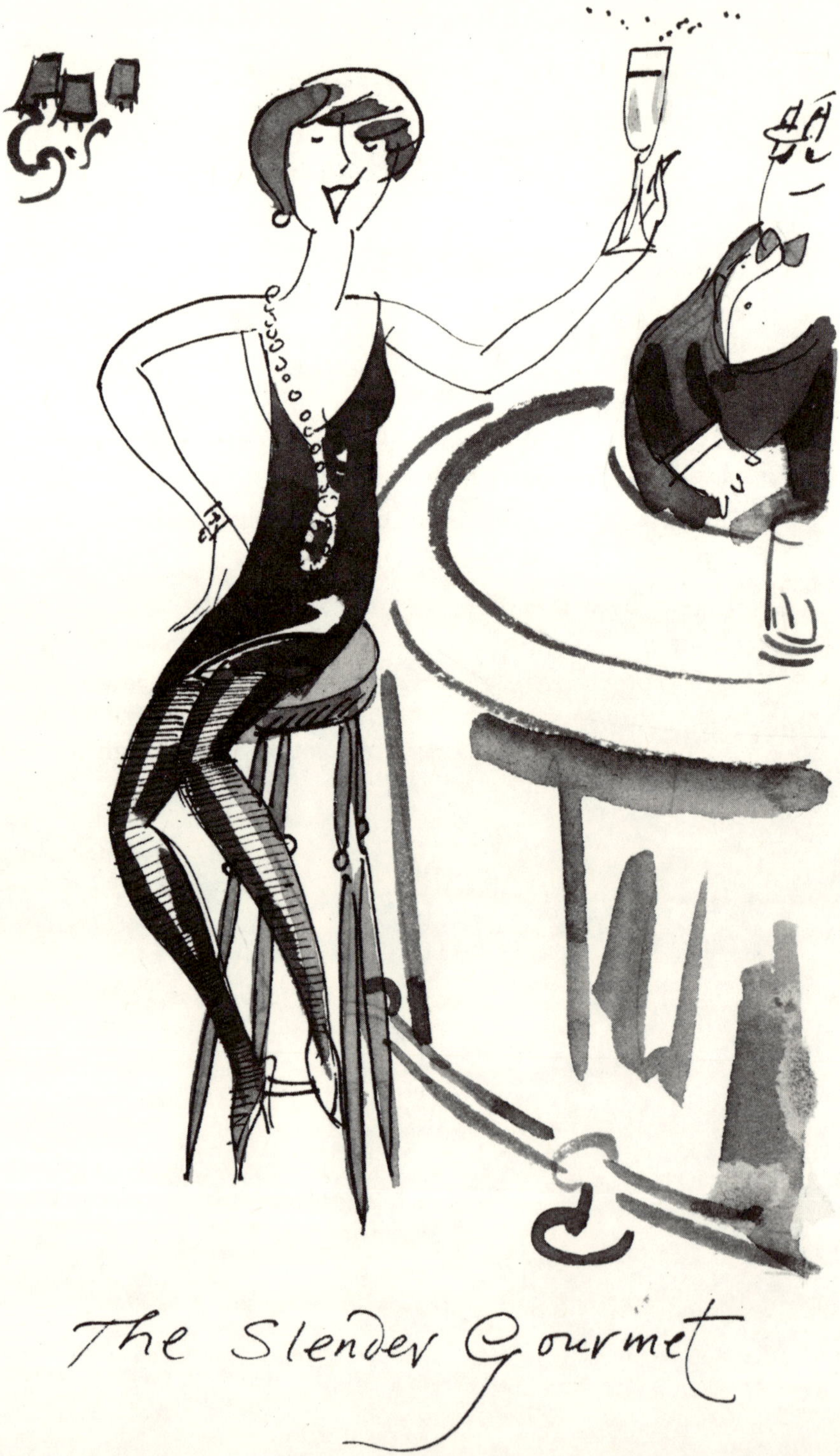

The Slender Gourmet

Introduction

The telephone rang in my studio one afternoon last summer and a distinctive, dancing voice announced itself to be that of Miss Joan Oliphant-Fraser. The name, worthy of any cartoonist's imagination, at once intrigued me. It was followed by the startling statement she had written a book to be entitled 'The Champagne Diet'. Once I had digested that, though not the Champagne as yet, we agreed to meet soon in my eyrie over Shaftesbury Avenue.

A stylish slender lady arrived, exuding vitality, clasping an equally slender MS and a promising looking parcel, that, unravelled, turned out to contain a chilled bottle of Roederer. This was to be the first of several stimulating meetings at the studio, Bracewell's, Maxim's, the Wine Cellar of Fortnums and her tiny flat near Curzon Street.

Bubbles burst, we danced divinely, exchanged ideas for the drawings and the odd variation in the text. I suspect the result is as uncoventional as the title, balancing Joan Oliphant-Fraser's liberated conception of the high life with a perfectly painless regimen for not letting it get the better of you.

We remain boon companions and hope the experience will benefit both the reader's palate and physique.

Michael ffolkes

Foreword

The Slender Gourmet Introduces the Champagne Lifestyle

You may well ask, 'Who is the Slender Gourmet' – an apparent contradiction in terms? A sylph? A bon viveur? Both, of course. It is possible and, more important, desirable to have one's gateaux and dance all night.

I have marvellous news for the young in heart, if not in calendar years. Born in a good vintage myself, I conduct a class in Yoga and Aerobics and eat like a filly.

Before I became The Slender Gourmet I was a dancer whose love of the good life was making me less than sylph-like. As I pirouetted to romantic nocturnes by Chopin and gazed into my partner's eyes, visions of little woodcock simmering in rich cream sauces, flambéed with Armagnac, or Crêpes filled with apples soaked in Calvados topped with country fresh clotted cream flashed through my mind.

Like others, I rebelled against the austerity and boredom of dieting and regimented press-ups. I was searching for a pleasurable way to lose a few pounds.

So I studied nutrition and certain facts emerged: a gourmet lifestyle could still be followed provided one observed certain rules which, far from detracting, actually enhance the pleasures of the table.

Not just a glass of bubbles

Champagne has always been my favourite wine. I drank it for breakfast on my sixteenth birthday and I have done so ever since. Then I discovered that it can become part of a successful slimming campaign which includes dining at the best restaurants or preparing special Slender Gourmet dishes at home.

I also decided that the exercises had to reflect the quality of this Champagne lifestyle. They too had to be fun and imaginative and, above all, done in comfortable, pleasing surroundings. Even a mildly vigorous work-out in a Gym should be followed by luxuriating in a jacuzzi letting the bubbles pummel away. To be even more imaginative, taking a trip in a hot-air balloon provides an opportunity of breathing deeply of fresh air that helps wonderfully to restore one's joie de vivre.

I have written the Champagne Diet for those of us who have acquired through success, excess or distress a few extra pounds. If you decide to follow this new Epicurean approach to dieting and exercising, not only will you become more lissom and enjoy better health and vitality but a whole new series of interests will evolve.

1 *A Little Overweight perhaps?*

One morning take a good look at yourself in a full-length mirror. The reflection that half-smiles back is not bad. In fact you could be described as well dressed, but what is *this* that spoils the line of your clothes? It wasn't there when you were twenty. What has happed in the intervening years? You have become successful; in short, too much food and, worse still, too many drinks.

The majority of us are not teetotallers; we drink convivially in wine bars, at lunchtime and with the evening meal. We drink not only when we are thirsty but in order to enjoy ourselves.

A mixture of liquid passes our lips throughout the day and evening ranging from whisky and sodas, gin and tonics, brandy, sherry, port, beer and carbohydrate laden cocktails like pinacoladas, cobblers and punches, not to mention carbonated fruit drinks, all of which can be high in artificial additives and unhealthy sugars.

What we drink is even more fattening that what we eat. If you were to write down every single drink you have during the day it could tot up to an amazing 1,000 calories plus!

Don't Give It Up!

Don't become abstemious – it's bad for the mental equilibrium as well as putting a damper on your life-style. Instead, be selective, keep to one drink only during your dieting period and let that drink be the very best, the Charlemagne of drinks, Champagne.

One other drink is an important accessory to the diet and that is the Champagne Companion, *Aqua Minerale*, which makes the bubbles go further.

Bottled water that comes from natural springs and spas contains lots of healthy minerals and is very different from tap water, which is not only deficient in minerals but can contain small deposits of arsenic. Though a little poison does you good occasionally, acting as a stimulant, it is not part of the Champagne Diet, which has its roots in wholesomeness. As Louis Pasteur, biologist and chemist said, 'Wine is the healthiest of drinks'. Why? Because a pure, unadulterated wine, like Champagne, contains vitamins, minerals, acids and enzymes that keep gourmets healthy and slender. These acids and enzymes also aid the digestion and thorough assimilation of food, preventing it from building up as deposits of fat in the body.

Champagne is perfect as an apéritif. It prepares the gastric juices for the meal ahead. During the meal it helps the metabolism of fats and tranquilizes the digestive system afterwards.

The Champagne Style of Dieting

Champagne contains only 75 calories to a 4 fl. oz glass and the Champagne Companion is calorie free.

When you follow the dietary ratio of 60% water to 40% Champagne, and assuming you might be drinking ten glasses a day, four glasses of Champagne and six of *Aqua Minerale* total only 300 calories, whereas ten assorted drinks could go well over 1,000 leaving you hardly any calories over for the Slender Gourmet style food which is a vital part of the Champagne Diet.

The Slender Gourmet Style of Eating

Food must be of the best. Simple fare like caviar, oysters, smoked salmon, filet steak and asparagus tips are all slimming and nutritious.

Meat pies, french fries, peas or puddings and breakfast of fried eggs and bacon are out on the grounds of being plebeian, fatty, carbohydrate and calorie loaded.

Every meal, whether eaten at home or at one of The Slender Gourmet recommended restaurants must match the excellence of Champagne. The Slender Gourmet's style of eating is a gastronomic adventure.

The Slender Gourmet Style of Exercising

The exercises must be both effective and fun. They can be the result of a leisure pursuit or become a part of your everyday round of activities.

The Champagne style of eating and drinking takes care of the pounds (even stones) and the Slender Gourmet exercises look after the inches.

2 *I Get a Kick from Champagne*

A glass or two of Champagne produces exhilaration without deflation. This is because the bubbles carry the alcohol into the blood stream more quickly than still wines or other drinks. We all need these stimuli, especially if we hit the dietary doldrums.

Cole Porter tried to make us believe he got no kick from Champagne. Quite false, he drank gallons and was just saying that to some lady who thrilled him even more.

What makes Champagne so special?

There is an abundance of sparkling wines on the market but they are not Champagne. The only sparkling wine that can call itself Champagne comes from a small region in the north-east of France around the mountain of Rheims and the Marne Valley stretching south down the Cotes des Blancs. It is here that everything comes together, soil, climate, grape varieties, skill and expertise of the vigneron and Mâitre de Cuvée to produce a great, pure wine.

Grape Varieties

Champagne, although a white wine, is made from both black and white grapes. Three varieties are used which contribute to its character. The Pinot Noir grape gives body and strength; Pinot Meunier, another black grape, gives freshness and youth; Chardonnay, a white grape, contributes finesse and elegance.

Non-Vintage for Everyday Drinking

For everyday drinking non-vintage Champagnes are the most popular, expressing the personality of the Houses that make them. You can expect a consistency of standard and style from year to year. Most Houses refer to their non-vintage as 'Brut' which mean extremely dry.

The best of the Grandes Marques (literally translated as 'big blends') are:

Perrier-Jouët, Louis Roederer, G. H. Mumm, Dry Monopole, Piper Heidsieck, Taittinger, Laurent-Perrier and Henriot.

It's a matter of taste whether you prefer a soft, light style like Mumm's Cordon Rouge to a bigger wine like Louis Roederer's Brut Premier which has a lot of character and depth for a non-vintage.

Pink Champagne or Rosé

Rosé Champagnes get their colour either from a small addition of still red wine or by leaving the skins of the black Pinot Noir grapes in contact with the 'must' (unfermented grape juice) for a short time.

A young Rosé can be light, fresh, a touch insouciant – perfect for an early morning encounter, whereas, a Rosé that has had a few years in a bottle can mature into a great Champagne with lots of body, fruitiness and character.

In spite of its slightly frivolous image, partly created by film stars of the Twenties, who used it as a bubble bath, Rosé or Pink Champagnes should be taken seriously.

Vintage for Special Occasions

A vintage is only declared in exceptionally good years when the grapes are of a high quality and the Champagne expresses the characteristics of that particular year.

For example, the Laurent Perrier '78 vintage was rounder, richer, more masculine perhaps, than the flowery, fragrant crisp '79.

de Luxe Champagnes

These Crême de la Crême Champagnes are made from the first pressings of the finest grapes.

Apart from the famous Dom Perignon, there are the equally prestigious Laurent Perrier 'Grand Siècle', Louis Roederer 'Cristal', G. H. Mumm 'René Lalou', Heidsieck Dry Monopole 'Diamant Bleu', Taittinger 'Comtes de Champagne', Piper Heidsieck 'Rare', Henriot 'Baccarat', Perrier-Jouët 'Belle Époque.'

When you have become a successful Slender Gourmet, reward yourself with one of these exceptional Champagnes.

The Slimmer's Champagne (The Ultra Brut)

Quietly, unobtrusively, without a big fanfare two Champagne Houses have produced a new style of Champagne which, being completely **SUGAR FREE**, is ideal for slimmers.

It was originally created at the request of jockeys and polo players who have to keep their weight down to a shadow of our more indulgent selves. After a race or match they need either to celebrate or commiserate. In each case, the occasion calls for Champagne.

A horse lover, maintaining that what was good enough for him was good enough for his horse, used to give his steed a tankard of Black Velvet – Guinness and Champagne! A Derby winner, perhaps!

A Slender Gourmet needs to be revived occasionally with the Slimmer's Special, the carbohydrate free, bone-dry type of Champagne.

There is a choice between Laurent-Perrier's Ultra Brut and Piper Heidsieck's Brut Sauvage. Brut Sauvage is a vintage whereas Ultra Brut is a blend of several vintages. Both are excellent; it's a matter of taste which you prefer. Try both to find out.

So Wickedly Delightful

The most popular Champagne in England today is the Brut, but sweet, or Demi-sec Champagnes are still obtainable. Although, as you might have guessed, they are not recommended for Aspiring Slender Gourmets.

Sweet wines were popular during the reign of Louis XV when a much sweeter style of Champagne was preferred. The wide-brimmed saucer glass was originally designed for this full-bodied aromatic wine, into which, the ladies of the court would dip slices of Madeira cake. But, they were not worried about weight. The curvaceous hourglass figure was fashionable and the gentlemen too relied on corsets to hold their manly shapes together.

There may be times, however, when your blood sugar is low and a glass of demi-sec revitalizes the system. If this is the case, Heidsieck Dry Monopole's 'Top Rich' is sweet without being cioying and would marry well with a simple plate of fraises du bois.

Look and Listen – Nose and Taste

When you hold a glass of Champagne up to the light its colour will range from pale straw (suggesting youth) to the golden tones of maturity.

Some people hold the glass to their ear. Cyril Ray, a renowned bon viveur, said 'a great Champagne speaks to you in its bubbles'. 'La Mousse', or the sparkle, consists of a lively flow that delicately explode with a small plop when they reach the surface of the wine, indicating a Champagne of elegance. Should they explode with a noisy pop, dissipate and subside flatly, this could indicate a young, brash wine of little breeding.

The bouquet which you received by nosing the wine, should be fresh and clean, veering towards flowery, fruity aromas.

Often the smell of the wine will be an indicator as to its taste, which should be dry, clean and pleasing. Nuances of flavour ranging from light, crisp, delicate, fruity, full, fragrant will come through, but always there is that refreshing tingle on the tongue that makes Champagne so aristocratic.

A great Champagne will have character, length (extension of flavour) and an aftertaste that lingers on the palate, and, if you are lucky, will remain after the wine is finished.

The Gods on Olympus only had nectar. We mortals are more fortunate in having Champagne.

The Champagne Library

For the Champagne connoisseur there is a diverting refresher course at Fortnum and Mason. Instead of books, bottles line the shelves of their Champagne Library which houses a collection of over sixty-five different premier Champagnes. These range in quality from non-vintage to rare vintage collections, as well as Cuvée Prestiges which are presented in beautiful bottles. One of the loveliest is Perrier-Jouët's 'Belle Epoque'. Garlanded with enamel hand-painted flowers that are fired directly on to the glass, the bottle was designed by Emile Galle in 1902 and is a perfect example of Art Nouveau. Today, in fact, empty magnums of Belle Époque can fetch almost as much money in the flea markets of Paris as the full standard size bottles filled with Champagne!

First Editions

Taittinger recently started a Designer series of labels drawn by famous artists. The first one, which commemorated the '78 vintage, was an abstract by Hungarian artist Victor Vasarely.

The second (current) edition is by the French painter Arman who designed a pattern of interlacing violins on a black lacquered background, symbolizing a

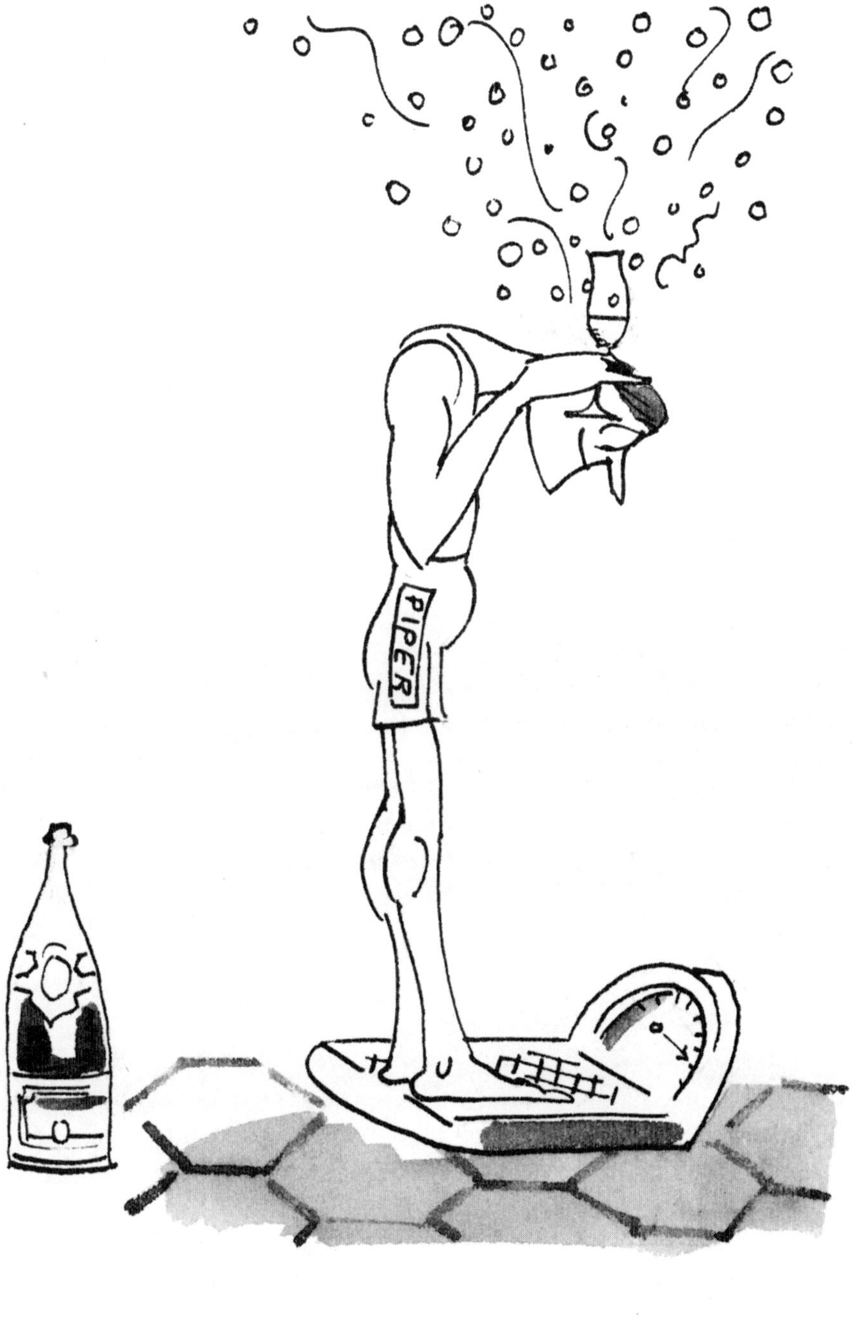

bone dry style of bubbly

Muse serenading the liquid stars of Champagne. This bottle contains their 1981 vintage, one of the smallest harvests since the War but of excellent quality.

Browsing through the bottles to decide which Champagne should accompany your evening meal is fun. If you are planning a small party a magnum (two bottles) is an economy. When empty, it will either make a door stop or, filled with bath salts, a stylish accessory.

Rare Editions

Many of the great Cuvées come in the same antique-shaped bottles as were originally commissioned by monarchs and potentates who ordered them in former times.

A bottle with a particularly lovely shape is Laurent-Perrier's 'Grand Siècle', a copy of the original bottle blown by the Master Glassblowers in the reign of The Sun King, Louis XIV.

Bumper Editions

A formidable bottle is the gigantic Nebuchadnezzar which holds the equivalent of twenty bottles.

One of Fortnum and Mason's elegant, tail-coated assistants, in gallant Herculean style, lifted it down from its pedestal for me to examine, explaining that in order to extract the cork, the bottle has to be placed in a reclining position. This giant has just reappeared on the market after an absence of around seventy years when the glass factory received a direct hit during a bombing raid in the First World War. Piper Heidsieck have produced just ten of these and Fortnums have acquired one.

Conversational Door Stops

The giant-sized bottles – Jeroboams – two magnums or four bottles: Rehoboams – six bottles; Methuselahs – eight bottles; Salamanazars – twelve bottles; Balthazars – sixteen, make great door stops, giving one something stylish on which to stub a big toe, or better still, to make a startling entrance accompanied by a few rich epithets.

3 *The Slender Gourmet Guide to Healthy Eating*

Simple, pure natural foods not only keep you healthy but slender too. This daily eating plan consists of foods rich in fibres, low on fats, veering away from salt and cutting sugars to the minimum.

Meat, game, poultry and fish should come from animals that have followed the Slender Gourmet lifestyle and been allowed to enjoy their natural habitat, eating only the best foods and exercising to keep their weight down. Better to resemble a caribou than a plump partridge.

Grooming the Inner Gourmet

It is important to keep as beautiful and slender within as without but to achieve this a good proportion of fibre or 'roughage' in your diet is essential. Fibre is found in cereals, grains, nuts, fruit, vegetables and salads.

Bread is a high-fibre food providing it is made from wholemeal or wholewheat flour which contains the whole grain. Some gourmet bakers add chopped walnuts, celery and poppy seeds to their recipe which bolsters up the fibre content as well as providing additional flavour and an *al dente* bite.

Bread made from white flour has less flavour and little nutritional value. But worse still, because its texture is soft and aereated, it acts like blotting paper, swelling up with liquid in the stomach. A couple of slices can leave you feeling and looking like the Michelin man for hours.

However, there is an exception – the long, French loaf familiar to us all tucked under the arm of a Parisian bicyclist. The crust compliment cheese, pâtes and breakfast-time marmalade. We know that Aborigines stimulate and massage their gums with twigs. This has a comparable effect. The soft, white centre must be discarded at all costs.

Pasta can help you slim

This is good news for devotees of spaghetti, noodles and rice. Wild rice, the seeds of which come from rare exotic grasses that grow in faraway swamps, is the In Pasta on the Slender Gourmet's Diet. Its distinctive texture and taste mixes well with the brown variety. Other sources of fibre are vegetables, fruit and salads.

A haute-cuisine potato

Do eat potatoes, but, as they have a high starch content, eat them in either of these two Slender Gourmet ways.

Bake the potatoes in their jackets, eat mainly the skins which contain most of the flavour and all the nutrients and discard the white starch in the middle, which birds adore.

Alternatively, Pommes Soufflées, potato balls, hollow in the centre, hot and crisp on the outside, are considered by many gourmets to be the quintessential potato.

Exotic fruit enzymes

Exotic fruits like mango, pineapple, paw paw and passion fruit contain acids and enzymes. When marinated or cooked with pork, beef and other meats and poultry they help to destroy the toxics and fats in the meat's tissues. Sometimes choose recipes or dishes that combine fruit with meats.

Citrus fruit such as lemons, grapefruits or oranges, though acid-tasting in the mouth, are alkaline in the stomach, and are particularly refreshing first thing in the morning when the body's alkaline level is low.

Lock up your lettuces

Both rabbits and gourmets can be forgiven for running away with members of the lettuce family, especially the interestingly leafed variety – the Autumn-tinged oak leaf, lamb's tongue, curly endive, crunchy red radicchio, tender spinach leaves, sorrel, spicy watercress and nasturtium leaves. A few of these leaves add verve to the standard Cos, Iceberg or hothouse lettuce-based salad.

Facts about fats

Too much fat can raise one's cholesterol level and clog up the arteries, ultimately leading to heart problems.

However, a certain amount of fat is needed to help protect the body's vital organs and to provide body heat and energy.

Make a point of eating less fat, especially saturated animal fats, so spread the butter sparingly on your bread and for weight loss use a low-fat spread which contains half the calories found in either butter or margerine.

Dress Up your Salad

With of course, only the very best olive, walnut or hazelnut oil. The first pressings or extra extra Virgin oils that come from France and Italy are best. Olive oil is popular in Mediterrean countries where, it is worth noting, heart disease incidence is very low. Use an equally good quality wine vinegar for your dressing. Some vinegars, like fine Champagnes, are produced only in exceptional years and are at their best when they have some bottle age, perhaps even fifty years. Otherwise, choose a white wine vinegar made from the elegant Chardonnay Champagne grape.

The merest 'pinch'

Too much salt (according to the experts we are all offenders) leads to high blood pressure. Refined salt, like refined flour, is not part of this Diet, but a little Rock or Sea salt is permitted. This contains iodine that stimulates the thyroid gland, which in turn helps the metabolism to function efficiently.

A cause of fatness can be too much salt in the diet, which leads to water retention. By cutting down on salt you could help the pounds diminish too.

However, gourmets and cooks need to use salt sometimes to bring out the flavour of certain foods. In this case, taste before you sprinkle and you may find you don't need any at all. Try flavouring food with alternative herbs and spices. Lemon juice for example, is a good substitute for salt with meat, poultry and fish.

The Salt Balancer

You can balance the sodium (it's the sodium in salt that's bad) with potassium.

Potassium is found in citrus fruits, figs, bananas, watercress, green peppers, meat, fish and grains.

If you are overly fond of salt, eat plenty of watercress with your meals or have a sliced banana, a fruit very high in potassium, with your breakfast cereal.

Your aim is to gradually reduce your salt intake to the merest 'pinch'.

To sin is to take sugar

Apart from ruining your teeth and bringing you out in spots, sugar-rich foods are the ones that can make you ideal casting for Grand Opera. Sugar is not a food as it has no nutritional value. Whenever possible fruit or dried fruit should be substituted for sugar and when you feel in need of a quick energy boost take a handful of grapes or whatever fruit is available.

For that morning bite

In spite of its sugar content, marmalade made from bitter Seville oranges that have had the white pith left on the skin has a 'wake you up' tang, freshens the taste-buds and the acids in the pith clean the teeth more effectively than many a toothpaste. Unfortunately, it is only home-made marmalade that has these dual qualities so buy the best Seville orange marmalade you can find to spread on your wholemeal toast. The Spanish onion has a different effect!

For Gourmets with a Sweet Tooth

Every diet must have its delectation, which need not be its downfall. On this diet it is chocolate, dark, plain and bitter, either thinly sculptured into shapes that act as containers for fruits, mousses, sorbets or parfaits, or on its own.

Be seduced by a super chocolate but not before 9 p.m. Chocolate is an indulgence and you mustn't be tempted until after the evening meal and then by a mint or mocha-flavoured stick or a Champagne truffle (70 calories a fling). The very best chocolates contain over 50% cacao which more than redeems the sinful sugar content because cacao induces a blissful state of utter contentment, a state in which you might find yourself murmuring to yourself, 'I love you, I think you're beautiful'.

Nearly all quality chocolates contain lecithin which is a nutrient derived from the Soya bean. Apart from helping to burn up fats it also keeps the body fats moving so that they don't settle in susceptible areas.

Is it food or an explosive?

You could be forgiven for wondering when the contents on the label lists such items as Crumbs with Colour E102, or antioxidant E30, Gelling Agents E401, Caseinate, Emulsifiers E472b, Fumaric Acid and a stabilizer. Your stomach would need a stabilizer if you were to eat this kind of convenience food.

Much better to keep to recognizable nourishment like fish, oysters and caviar.

Some of the best fish in the world, sole, hake and halibut, come from the cold, North Atlantic waters. Meanwhile, the King of fish, the wild salmon, spends a lot of its life in the rivers, swimming and leaping upstream in an effort to get back to its breeding grounds. This leaping and swimming upstream keeps it slender, giving it more taste and less fat than the salmon reared in peaceful Highland lochs.

Fish is an excellent source of protein, low in saturated fat, besides containing vital minerals like calcium and phosphorous.

Crustaceans

A Champagne Diet would be incomplete without oysters, lobsters and giant-sized Dublin Bay Prawns, alias French Langoustine and Italian Scampi.

An oyster is only five calories and full of rejuvenating protein; besides being a rich source of phosphorous salts, chalk, iron, copper, manganese and a high proportion of iodine, it also contains vitamins A, B1, C and D.

Apart from being a food it is regarded as a beauty treatment, restoring water content to the skin and lessening facial lines and wrinkles, but its greatest claim to fame is that it may be an aphrodisiac.

Lobster meat and deshelled prawns are only thirty calories an ounce of concentrated protein. Protein clings to the ribs which is why small portions go further.

Caviar for glamour

Eggs, whether they come from cod, plaice, sole or any other fish, have exceptional nutritional value, but the most glamorous roe comes from the female sturgeon – caviar. Only seventy-five calories an ounze, it is a perfectly balanced food containing 30% protein, 16% polyunsaturated fish fat and 4% minerals; the rest is water.

Happy Beef

A lot of meat comes from animals which are mass reared. They are injected with hormones to plump them up and since penned cattle are easy prey to illness and disease, they are regularly injected with antibiotics to kill any germs. When we eat meat raised in these conditions we consume hormones and antibiotics retained in the meat's fatty tissues.

You are more likely to avoid this by eating quality meat from animals which have been allowed to graze on pastureland rather than having been cooped up in unhealthy battery conditions.

The best beef is the Scottish Black Angus, or the Charolias from France, In Japan, the prize cattle are particularly well-looked-after, getting a daily hand massage to ensure tender steaks. People are treated with less sensitivity.

Wild venison, hare and rabbit or birds like pheasant and duck which have also missed the hypodermic needle are low on fat because they have been running or flying around and have lots of flavour from grazing on sweet meadow grass and nibbling the tops of herb-flavoured hedges.

The hi-fibrous Bird

Chicken is a particularly good food for slimmers as it is low in fats yet high in protein. Again, you need to avoid battery reared birds that have been raised on cheap fish meal. Look for free-range chickens which have led happy lives strutting and clucking around a farmyard while waiting to be fed their hi-fibre diet of maze, corn and milk.

DO's and DONT's of Dieting

DO: Eat slowly. Champagne slows down your eating speed. In order to pick up your glass you have to put down your knife and fork. This reduces your eating speed to a gentle 'cruising' pace. By thoroughly masticating your food and extracting every nuance of texture and taste you'll find that you need less to satisfy your appetite.

DO: Eat less bread. Use a sharp knife and cut your wholemeal bread in wafer-thin slices.

DO: Use less salt; taste before you sprinkle.

DO: Have skimmed milk in tea or coffee; it has approximately half the fat content of other milks in spite of being just as rich in protein and calcium. You need calcium for bone maintenance.

DON'T: Eat fried foods. When the pan requires greasing use a quality oil instead of butter, or a non-stick pan.

DON'T: Take sugar in tea or coffee: don't even keep any in the house. Keep one pot of the best honey for your breakfast cereal, but try, if possible, to replace the honey with natural fruit sugars which are found in all fresh and dried fruits.

DON'T: Above all else, become a calorie counter, they are such dreary bores. You'll find that by cutting down on fats, sugars especially, white starches and eating smaller portions of food, and eating slowly, your calorie intake will diminish anyway.

4 *How to Follow the Champagne Diet*

'I am drinking stars' exclaimed the monk in rapturous tones as he took his first sip of Champagne.

'Drinking stars' is the lift that a diet needs to drag it away from the grapefruit and lettuce doldrums and make it a success. The reason why so many diets fail is because they are based on the self-denial principal: 'Can't do this', 'Mustn't have that' and similar dull repetitions.

This diet works because it has style and is glamorous besides being slimming and healthy.

When to Drink Champagne and How Much

This might be your first question and who better to answer it than Madame Bollinger who said, 'I drink it when I'm happy and when I'm sad. Sometimes I drink it when I'm alone. When I have company I consider it obligatory. I trifle with it if I'm not hungry and drink it when I am. Otherwise, I never touch it – unless I'm thirsty.'

This pretty well covers all possibilities. However, on the diet restraint is necessary. Aim for around three or four glasses a day, so you may decide to miss a glass at lunchtime prefering to have an early evening apéritif followed by a couple of glasses during dinner and one instead of a liqueur or port at the end. There could be emergency situations, however. For example:

Do You Flag at 11(am)?

Perhaps you are suffering from a shortage of Pink. Colour affects our moods and emotions. Picasso had his 'blue' period, white is spiritual, black sombre, pastel shades soothe, whereas red incites the passions. To view life through 'pink-tinted' spectacles is a philosophical way of seeing things at their rosiest. Looking at pink, especially when it sparkles, is in a glass and called Taittinger Comtes de Champagne lifts the morale up to Cloud Nine. Strangely enough, golden hued Champagne doesn't have quite that effect in the morning; it must be the colour that counts.

For Those Stressful Moments

Instead of swallowing pills, take your minerals and vitamins the natural way; drink a glass of Champagne.

Pure quality wines contain mineral salts such as potassium, iron, calcium and magnesium, plus water-soluble vitamins C and B complex, according to Dr Maury in his book '*Wine is the Best Medicine*'.

For those days that seem more fateful than others try this Mimosa Cocktail. Whisk a raw egg yolk (protein and lecithin) with freshly squeezed orange juice (vitamin C) and top up with Champagne.

Become a Two-Handed Drinker

As part of the diet don't forget the Champagne Companion. Make it a habit to match each glass of Champagne with a glass and a half of mineral water. There is something very reassuring about having two glasses on the go. Sip the Champagne and swallow the water. If you are in the middle of an animated conversation you are not always aware of what you are drinking anyway. On those occasions reach for the water and save the bubbles for the lull when you can give them your undivided attention.

You are attempting to drink a ratio of approximately 60% water to 40% Champagne, but if it occasionally gets closer to 50% – 50% don't worry. Don't swing into reverse though and drink more Champagne than water.

How Much Weight to Lose

At the onset of your diet you need to decide how much weight you want to lose. As a general guideline, if you want to lose less than two stone cut down to between 1,300 and 1,500 calories a day. Don't rush, however, and try to lose two stone in two weeks. It probably took you month's, even years, to collect the surplus so don't try or expect to be unencumbered in a fortnight.

Aim to lose eight to twelve pounds in four weeks. It's a happy diet, so if you have to stay with it for another four to eight weeks it will not be a hardship.

For Extra Weight Loss

If after a week or so, the pound's won't move cut your calories to 900 to 1,000 a day for two or three days.

Indulge your whims

If the menu is very tempting, don't resist, eat and enjoy yourself (within reason), for tomorrow is another day when you *can* take care of the previous day's excesses. Perhaps you overdid it by 500 calories; that's all right, the balance can be adjusted during the forthcoming week. It's not your daily but your overall weekly intake that counts. This means you can eat and drink according to the social occasion and your lifestyle. For example, you had a marvellous seven-course banquet (small taste-provoking portions, naturally); the next morning you are not so hungry, so choose the low-calorie Slimmer's Special, followed at lunchtime with a small fish delicacy. By the evening you may be getting your appetite back so dine at home and prepare one of the special Slender Gourmet low-calorie dinners created by Chef Brian Steele.

The diet consists of three meals a day, breakfast, lunch and dinner. No snacks between meals.

A Prelude to the Day

Breakfast is important to start afresh and put the best fork forward. You can choose from one of three breakfasts depending on how hungry you feel, what you had to eat the previous evening and what your plans are for the day ahead.

The traditional bacon and eggs, white toast and sugary sweet marmalade washed down with coffee is OUT. It is too high in foods that form acids in the body. Over-acidity can lead to all sorts of minor and major complaints like indigestion, insatiable appetite, cellulitis and arthritis. Any of these conditions could turn you into a Failed Slender Gourmet and hobbling to your favourite bar stool is not the Champagne image.

Every morning it is important to re-establish the body's acid/alkaline balance. A healthy body needs to maintain a ratio of approximately 75% alkaline to 25% acid.

The following three breakfasts take care of this.

If you wake up feeling 'peckish' or have a long day ahead with the possibility of only a light lunch, then the Slender Gourmet Health Bowl is nourishing. It lines the stomach and keeps the hunger pangs at bay.

Breakfast No. 1 *The Slender Gourmet Health Bowl*

Make a mix from both the acid- and alkaline-forming foods on this list. Aim for three parts alkaline to one part acid.

Alkaline-forming foods	cals	Acid-forming foods	cals
½ carton natural yoghurt	30	Grains and cereals.	
Fresh or dried fruit:		2 tbsp. crunchy Muesli	
1 oz. berries	8	including a sprinkling of	
½ apple	7	seeds like sunflower,	
small peach or pear	30	pumpkin, sesame	200
5 dried apricots or hunzas	50		
(soaked overnight)		Tsp. honey (optional)	30

Oh, that this too solid flesh would melt . . . Hamlet didn't know, but if you want to help the body burn up surplus fats, sprinkle Lecithin granules over your Muesli. Remember what I said about Lecithin in the chapter on Healthy Eating.

Breakfast No. 2 *The Continental*

Presentation is everything. A large tray covered with a white linen cloth on which reposes a class of chilled, freshly squeezed (only minutes before) orange juice, thinly sliced wholemeal toast aereating in a silver toast rack, and a jar of marmalade made from Seville oranges. This should be accompanied by a pot of china tea (less caffeine content than Indian) – either a Lapsang Souchong which has delicate, smoky overtones or Green Gunpowder which, far from being explosive, is practically caffeine free. If you prefer coffee with your breakfast choose a de-caffinated variety.

A perfect flower in a vase provides food for the soul, while a copy of *The Times* provides something for the brain. Definitely a breakfast to linger over.

Breakfast No. 3 *The Slimmer's Special*

If you had a rather splendid meal the previous evening, you might need to economize on your calories, so half a pink grapefruit (30 calories) and a cup of Mint tea made from fresh mint leaves.

A Little Midday Sustenance

Lunch should be light, nutritious and sustaining. Oysters, caviar, giant prawns, lobster, crab, smoked salmon are all low-calorie, high-protein foods. Eaten with a green salad or vegetables they provide all the nutrition your body needs to carry you over until the dinner gong.

A simple lunch at home might be:

2 or 3 giant prawns (if you are not too squeamish do suck the prawn's head, it's tasty and rich in minerals.)

2 or 3 little mouth-size quail's eggs.

Unlimited sprigs of watercress, lemon juice and pepper.

2 wafer-thin slices of wholemeal bread covered with the merest scrape of butter.

Fruit in season or a slice of melon.

Otherwise eat at one of the Champagne, Caviar and Oyster Bars listed in Chapter 6.

The Moon Rises

The day builds up to the evening meal when there is time to sit down, either at home or in a restaurant, so why not make it the entire evening's entertainment?

5 *Following the Champagne Diet at Home*

A Chef's Lament

'My poor body, heavy with the residue of so many rich and delectable sauces, was so well covered that it weighed me to the ground and around my waist the centimetres crept, covering a considerable distance,' lamented Michel Guérard, a very fat Chef. Deciding to do something about his weight problem, he went to a Health Farm, where he reported receiving 'a sharp blow in the taste buds'. After eating what seemed like endless acres of undressed lettuce leaves and grated carrots, he emerged many kilos lighter but bordering on despair, 'unable' he said 'to feel the vibrations that made his eye, nose, palate and touch sing when a really successful dish appeared'. He felt isolated, cut off, surrounded by a closing wall of frustration. Out of this despair developed a resolve to create a new style of cooking which would appeal to people who love to eat but want to lose weight.

He experimented with new ways of cooking using very little fat and no flour or sugar and achieved a much lighter style of cuisine which he called Cuisine Minceur.

Cuisine Minceur is delicious but requires a lot of preparation and expertise. I was looking instead for a similar, but simpler form of gourmet cooking which could be prepared easily and with the minimum of time and at home.

I then met Brian Steele, Chef du Cuisine at the Holiday Inn's Flagship Hotel at Swiss Cottage and a member of the elite 'Society of Master Chefs' and asked him if he would create some menus for the Champage Diet, seven starters, seven main courses and seven desserts so that one from each group could be chosen to form a three-course meal.

These recipes, like Michel Guérard's 'Cuisine Minceur', are based on low animal fats, flour, salt and no refined white sugar. For sweetening Brian used fruit purées, fructose or liqueur. Fructose is a fruit derivative and contains half the calories of sugar.

Here are the Recipes:

Recipes Created by Master Chef Brian Steele

Starter	*Main Course*	*Dessert*
Covent Garden Quiche	Salmon en Papillote	Jamaican Fruit Salad
Gravad Lax	Veal Cutlet in a Green Waistcoat	Bananas en Papillote
Chicken Liver Gateaux	Paupiette of Sole with Spinach	Champagne Zabaglione
Prawn and French Bean Salad	Pork Fillet Diable	Royal Kir Sorbet
Melon Malibu	Scampi Pernod and Wild Rice	Caramelised Oranges
Oysters in Champagne Sauce	Chicken Mango coated in coconut	Kiwi Surprise
Asparagus with Orange Sabayon	Surf and Turf	Tarte aux Abricots

Serve the main course with fresh vegetables in season and/or a salad.

All recipes, unless otherwise stated, are for two people.

Covent Garden Quiche

6 – 8 crisp green cabbage leaves
50 g (2 oz) finely chopped onion
25 g (1 oz) diced red pepper
50 g (2 oz) sliced button mushrooms
5 ml (1 teasp.) chopped chives
Pinch of basil & thyme
Ground pepper & sea salt
125 ml (¼ pt) skimmed milk
1 egg

1) Set oven to gas mark 7 (220°C, 425°F)
2) Remove the thick stalk from the cabbage leaves. Place the leaves in boiling water for 4 mins and then into cold water (blanching). Allow to drain.
3) Gently heat a non-stick saucepan and add the onion, pepper, sliced mushrooms and herbs.
4) Stir constantly to prevent sticking until the mushrooms exude their juice. Continue cooking until the juice has evaporated. Allow to cool.
5) Beat the egg & milk together, season with salt and pepper.
6) Add the cooked mixture to the egg mix.
7) Line two 10 cm (4 inch) individual moulds or quiche tins with the cabbage leaves.
8) Pour in the mixture, cover with a circle of cabbage leaf and fold over the outer leaves to enclose the filling.
9) Cover with tin foil and bake in a water bath for 15 – 20 minutes. Allow to set for 5 minutes before turning out.

Salmon en Papillote with Champagne and Leeks (For the Love of Slimming)

Two 150 g (6 oz) skinned salmon fillets
100 g (4 oz) finely shredded whites of leeks
125 ml (¼ pt) champagne
1 lemon (for garnish)
Juice of ½ lemon
10 tarragon leaves
Milled pepper and sea salt

1) Prepare four 30 cm (12 inch) square sheets of tin foil, folded in half (together) and draw the shape of half a heart. Cut out the shape which will give you four heart shapes.
2) Season the salmon fillets with the salt and pepper. Place each fillet on one piece of foil. Add the lemon juice.
3) Cook the shredded leeks in boiling water for 10 seconds and divide it between the fillets.
4) Add the tarragon leaves and pour on the champagne.
5) Place the other shape of foil on top of each heart and neatly fold all the edges together, ensuring the seal is tight and that the shape is maintained.
6) Cook on a baking sheet in a moderate over for 12 – 15 minutes at gas mark 6, (200°C, 400°F).
7) Serve with a tomato and chive salad.

Jamaican Fruit Salad

1 whole baby pineapple
1 lime
1 small paw paw
1 guava
One sixth of a gill of white rum

1) Cut the pineapple in half, lengthwise. Using a sharp knife, cut around the flesh and remove it peaving the shell behind.
2) Remove the core and discard.
3) Cut the pineapple into even pieces.
4) Peel and dice the paw paw and guava and mix it with the pineapple.
5) Cover with the rum and replace the mixture into the shells.
6) Decorate with sliced lime.

Gravad Lax

Two 75 – 100 g (3 – 4 oz) fresh salmon fillets
5 ml (1 teasp.) fruit sugar
5 ml (1 teasp.) ground sea salt
2.5 ml (½ teasp.) ground white pepper
40 ml (2 tablesp.) olive oil
Lemon for garnish
Bunch of fresh dill

1) Place one fillet, skin side down, in a dish.
2) Wash and chop the dill and sprinkle it over the fillet.
3) Blend the salt, pepper and sugar with the oil and spread onto the fillet.
4) Place the second fillet on top, skin uppermost, and wrap the fish in silver foil.
5) Place a board or plate on top with a heavy weight on it and place in the refrigerator for 3 days.
6) Unwrap the fish and scrape most of the dill away. Slice very thinly and serve with a wedge of lemon.

Grilled Veal Cutlet in a Green Waistcoat

Two 200 g (8 oz) veal cutlets
25 g (2 oz) chopped onions
50 g (4 oz) sliced mushrooms
8 large spinach leaves
Rosemary
Milled pepper/sea salt

1) Set oven to gas mark 7 (220°C, 425°F)
2) Season the veal cutlets and sprinkle with rosemary. Grill until nearly cooked.
3) Blanch the spinach leaves and drain. Cover a dinner plate with half of them.
4) In a non-stick pan heat the onions and mushrooms until the mushrooms exude their juice.
5) Place each cutlet in the centre of a plate covered with spinach.
6) Put half the mushrooms and onions onto each cutlet and fold the spinach over to form an envelope.
7) Place the parcels in an ovenproof dish, cover and cook for a further 10 minutes.

Bananas en Papillote

2 bananas
100 g (4 oz) apricot purée (hot)
4 mint leaves
5 cm (2 inches) cinnamon stick

1) Set the oven at a moderate temperature.
2) Peel the bananas and place each one in an oblong piece of tin foil, about 30 × 20 cm (12 × 8 inches).
3) Divide the apricot purée, mint leaves and cinnamon stick between the bananas and then seal the foil tightly.
4) Cook for 10 minutes and serve the bananas in their foil cases on a plate.

Chicken Liver Gateaux

100 g (4 oz) chicken livers
1 egg
125 ml (¼ pt) skimmed milk
½ clove pressure garlic
Pinch nutmeg
Milled pepper, ground sea salt
Chopped parsley

1) Place all the ingredients into a liquidiser and liquidise for 1 minute on a low speed.
2) Divide into 2 ramekin moulds which have been brushed with water. (Any sinew in the chicken livers will remain at the bottom of the liquidiser.)
3) Place in a shallow roasting tray and fill the tray with water so that it half-covers the moulds.
4) Cover with tin foil and bake in moderate oven for 30 minutes at gas mark 6 (200°C, 400°F). Prick the foil to enable the steam to escape after it has cooked.
5) The gateau may be served in the ramekins, hot or cold. If served cold it may be accompanied with wholemeal oat cakes and a little salad to decorate.

Paupiette of Sole with Spinach

Six 50 g (1½ – 2 oz) lemon sole fillets (black skin removed)
100 g (4 oz) cooked spinach
25 g (1 oz) finely chopped onion
125 ml (¼ pt) champagne
65 ml (⅛ pt) dry white wine (or vermouth)
Milled pepper, ground sea salt
Nutmeg
5 ml (1 teasp.) chopped parsley
2 egg yolks

1) Lay fillets of sole on a plate, skin side up. Season with sea salt and milled pepper.
2) Season the spinach with a pinch of nutmeg.
3) Divide the spinach evenly between the 6 fillets.
4) Fold the fillets in half, enveloping the spinach.
5) Place in a non-stick frying pan. Add the chopped onions, champagne and white wine. Cover with a lid.
6) Gently bring to the boil and simmer for 7 – 10 minutes. Remove the fillets and keep warm.
7) Allow the remaining stock to cool in the pan. Add the 2 yolks and parsley and whisk continuously over a small pan, a quarter filled with simmering water. The yolks should double in volume.
8) Care must be taken not to let the mixture cook too quickly over too hot a pan as this may result in scrambling the eggs.
9) Place the fillets on hot plates and mask with the sauce.

Champagne Zabaglione

2 egg yolks
80 ml (4 tablesp.) champagne
20 ml (1 tablesp.) fruit sugar
Grating of lemon peel

1) Put all the ingredients into the top of a double boiler and whisk together over steaming water. Do not allow to boil.
2) Whisk until the mixture has trebled in volume and is light and frothy.
3) Pour into warm glasses and serve immediately.

Prawn and French Bean Salad

200 g (8 oz) french beans
150 g (6 oz) prawns (fresh or frozen and thawed)
1 small head of red radicchio
Juice of 1 lime
6 mint leaves/chopped parsley
40 ml (2 tablesp.) wine vinegar dressing
60 ml (3 tablesp.) dry sherry
Milled pepper and sea salt

1) Top and tail the beans, wash and cook in boiling water for 5 – 6 minutes so they remain crisp. Place into cold water and drain.
2) Finely chop the mint and parsley and mix with the wine vinegar, sherry and lime juice.
3) Divide the radicchio into individual leaves, wash thoroughly and dry gently in a cloth.
4) Arrange the leaves on a plate and place the beans on the top in a neat bundle. Sprinkle over the prawns.
5) Season with the salt and pepper. Add the dressing as required.

Pork Fillet Diable

(with Raspberry Vinegar and Mustard Seed Sauce)

Two 150 g (6 oz) pork fillets
50 g (2 oz) finely chopped onion
200 g (2 oz) liquidized raspberries (fresh or frozen)
50 g (2 oz) raspberry vinegar
125 ml (¼ pt) unsweetened red grape juice
1 small eating apple
5 ml (1 teasp.) mustard seeds
Milled pepper & sea salt

1) Cut each fillet into 3 even lengths and flatten out. Season and grill until cooked. (About 10 minutes).
2) Meanwhile place the onions in a non-stick pan and add the vinegar. Bring it to the boil and reduce it to a third of its original volume.
3) Strain the raspberries to remove the pips and add to the pan with the grape juice and mustard seeds. Re-boil and simmer for 5 minutes.
4) Peel and core the apple, cut into quarters and slice into the sauce.
5) Place the fillets on serving plates and mask with the sauce.

Royal Kir Sorbet

(serves 4)

300 g (12 oz) blackcurrants (frozen or tinned)
(A mixture of blackcurrants and redcurrants may be used.)
500 ml (1 pt) water
50 g (2 oz) fruit sugar
40 ml (2 tablesp.) creme de cassis (optional)
Juice of ½ lemon
2 egg whites

1) Wash and pick the fruit.
2) Place in a saucepan with 60 ml (3 tablesp.) water. Bring to the boil and simmer until the fruit becomes pulpy. Liquidise and pour into a clean bowl. Allow to cool.
3) Add the lemon juice and creme de cassis.
4) Put the fruit, sugar and water into a pan and boil rapidly to a syrup. (To test: remove a little of the syrup and then pour it back into the pan; if ready it will form a long thread.)
5) Allow to cool.
6) Stir the syrup into the fruit purée and put it into a freezer tray. Freeze for an hour, stirring occasionally until it becomes mushy.
7) Beat the egg whites until they form soft peaks.
8) Fold the fruit pulp into the egg whites.
9) Turn into 2 small freezer containers and allow to freeze for up to 5 hours.

Note: It is advisable to remove the sorbet from the freezer about 45 minutes before it is served. It should be placed in a refrigerator where it will soften slightly.

Melon Malibu

1 Ogen melon
1 fresh mandarin
8 peeled lychees (fresh or tinned)
One sixth of a gill of Malibu

1) Cut the melon in half and remove the seeds.
2) Peel and segment the mandarin.
3) Mix the segments and lychees and place into the melon.
4) Moisten with the Malibu and serve chilled.

Scampi Pernod and Wild Rice

250 g (10 oz) peeled scampi
25 g (1 oz) finely chopped onions
160 ml (8 tablesp.) Pernod
125 ml (¼ pt) dry white wine
2 egg yolks
Milled pepper, ground sea salt
Tarragon leaves
2.5 ml (½ teasp.) chopped parsley

1) Place scampi and chopped onions in a non-stick frying pan and season.
2) Add the white wine and half the Pernod.
3) Bring to the boil and simmer for 3 – 4 minutes. Remove the scampi and keep it warm.
4) Reduce the cooking liquor to one-third of its original volume. Allow to cool in the frying pan.
5) Add the egg yolks, remaining Pernod, parsley and tarragon leaves. Whisk continuously over a small pan, a quarter filled with simmering water, until the mixture doubles its volume and thickens.
6) Place the scampi on a hot plate and mask with the sauce.

Wild Rice:

1) Wash 50 g (2 oz) wild rice in cold running water. Cover with ½ pt salted water.
2) Cover tightly and cook over a low heat for 45 minutes.

Caramalised Oranges

2 oranges
250 ml (½ pt) water
20 ml (1 tablesp.) fruit sugar
40 ml (2 tablesp.) orange liqueur
40 ml (2 tablesp.) Grenadine (optional)

1) Peel the oranges with a potato peeler and cut the skin into very thin strips.
2) Carefully remove the pith from the orange.
3) Slice the oranges thinly and place into a serving dish. Pour over the liqueur.
4) Boil the water and the sugar together and add the strips of rind. Continue boiling until a syrup is formed.
5) Remove from the heat, add the Grenadine and pour over the sliced oranges.
6) Allow to cool in a refrigerator.

Oysters in Champagne Sauce

12 oysters
160 ml (8 tablesp.) champagne
2 egg yolks
20 ml (1 tablesp.) water
Milled pepper

1) Open the oysters and remove them from their shells. Season with the pepper.
2) Strain their juice through a fine cloth.
3) Wash out the shells and put them onto an oyster dish (or plate) in a warm oven.
4) Boil the champagne and allow it to reduce to a quarter of its original volume.
5) Allow to cool and then whisk in the egg yolks over a small pan a quarter full of simmering water until the mixture doubles in volume and thickens. Remove from the heat.
6) Poach the oysters in their own juice for 30 seconds, drain and replace them in their shells.
7) Whisk the poaching liquid into the sauce.
8) Cover each oyster with sauce and place in a very hot oven until they turn golden brown. (2 – 3 minutes.)

Chicken Mango coated in Coconut

Two 150 g (6 oz) chicken supremes (skin removed)
75 g (3 oz) mango, cut into strips
Milled pepper and sea salt
Coating: 1 egg
25 g (1 oz) wholemeal flour
50 g (2 oz) desiccated coconut
10 g (½ oz) olive oil

1) Remove the chicken fillet from the breast and gently flatten the breast. Cut the breast lengthwise very carefully to form a pocket.
2) Stuff the pocket with the mango.
3) Replace the fillet and pat gently to form a seal. Season the chicken.
4) Beat the egg yolk with a little water. Dust the chicken breast with the flour, dip into the egg mixture and turn.
5) Coat both sides with the coconut.
6) Fry carefully in the olive oil till light golden brown. Place on a baking sheet and finish cooking in a moderate oven for 15 – 20 minutes at gas mark 6 (200°C, 400°F.)

Kiwi Surprise

3 kiwi fruit
125 g (5 oz) low fat natural yoghurt
Coarsely grated rind of an orange
Pinch ground ginger
2.5 ml (½ teasp.) pink peppercorns (optional)
Grand Marnier/orange curacao

1) Peel the kiwi fruit and slice. Arrange around the edge of the serving dishes.
2) Sprinkle with the liqueur.
3) Mix the orange rind, ginger and peppercorns into the yoghurt.
4) Pour this carefully into the centre of the fruit.
5) Chill and serve.

Asparagus with Orange Sabayon

12 medium asparagus spears
1 orange
1 egg yolk
8 fresh mint leaves, finely chopped
10 ml (2 teasps.) wine vinegar
Milled pepper, ground sea salt

1) Wash the asparagus and cut off the woody ends.
2) Tie into bundles with fine string and gently cook in boiling water until tender.
3) Place the egg yolk, wine vinegar and grated rind and juice of the orange into a bowl and whisk continuously over a small pan, a quarter full of simmering water (thus making a bain-marie or double saucepan.)
4) Whisk until the mixture doubles in volume and acquires a thick consistency. (The mixture may be removed from the hot water pan to prevent it getting too hot and scrambling.)
5) Add the freshly chopped mint and serve immediately.

Surf and Turf

250 g (10 oz) chicken supremes (skin removed)
150 g (6 oz) peeled scampi
100 g (4 oz) finely chopped onion
250 g (10 oz) fresh tomatoes
50 g (2 oz) diced green pepper
1 garlic clove (peeled and pressed)
125 ml (¼ pt) dry white wine
Milled pepper and sea salt
5 ml (teasp.) chopped basil
10 ml (2 teasp.) tomato puree

1) Cut the chicken into scampi-sized pieces.
2) Remove the core from the tomatoes and place them into boiling water for 10 seconds. Put straight into cold water and remove the skins.
3) Cut each tomato into 4 and remove the seeds and pulp. (This can be liquidized and strained into the sauce). Coarsely chop the remainder.
4) Place the chopped onions, garlic and peppers in a non-stick pan and cook gently for 2 minutes.
5) Add the wine and reduce by half. Add the tomato, liquidised pulp and tomato purée. Season and add the basil.
6) Cook for 8 – 10 minutes. Add the chicken and cook for 5 more minutes and finally the scampi for another 3 minutes.
7) Serve with wild rice.

Tarte aux Abricots

(serves four)

100 g (4 oz) wholemal flour
50 g (2 oz) polyunsaturated fat (eg Flora)
Pinch ground sea salt
Water to mix pastry and cook apples
5 ml (1 teasp.) lemon juice
125 g (5 oz) peeled, cored cooking apples
Pinch ground cinnamon
375 g (15 oz) tinned apricots (in natural juice)
2.5 ml (½ teasp.) fruit sugar
Glaze: 100 g (4 oz) dried, soaked apricots
10 ml (2 teasp.) apricot brandy
Juice from tinned apricots
Liquid from soaked apricots

1) Set oven to gas mark 7 (220°C, 425°F)
2) Rub the fat into the salt and flour. Put half the lemon juice into about ⅛ pt water and stir into the mixture to form the pastry. (Do not add too much water and thus make the pastry too wet.)
3) Allow to rest for 15 minutes.
4) Line an 18 cm (7 inch) flan ring and bake blind for 5 – 7 minutes so that the pastry sets.
5) Cook the apples with the rest of the lemon juice, cinnamon, sugar and enough water to form a purée. Spread this across the bottom of the flan and cook for another 10 – 15 minutes.
6) Arrange the tinned apricots over the apple.
7) Boil the dried apricots in their liquid and the juice from the tin until they form a pulp. (This may take about 30 minutes.) Liquidise for 30 seconds and add the brandy.
8) Pour over the apricots and allow to cool.

Note: The apricot purée will be enough for the Bananas en Papillote.

Dining at Home

Eating at home should be just as enjoyable as dining out. Invite a friend to dinner, set the scene, a candlelit table with the Champagne cooling in an ice bucket (filled with ice cubes and water). Everything should sparkle, the Champagne, the *pièce de resistance*, the conversation and the glassware. To do justice to Champagne the choice of glass is important; it should show off the colour and bubbles to best advantage. Make sure that you like the weight and feel of the glass in your hand, apart from its decorative appearance on the table.

Do you have a languishing mousse?

Choose the narrow flute or tall tulip rather than the open saucer type glass whose shape encourages the bubbles to dissipate. There is nothing more irksome than having repeatedly to top up your glass from the bottle in an effort to revive a languishing mousse.

Professor Claus Riedel, one of the great glassmakers, may have come up with the answer. After years of research he has evolved a technique whereby the glass not only holds the bubbles for a longer period of time but keeps them active as they leave the glass to settle on the tastebuds of the tongue, filling, as the Professor says 'our mouth with a festive tingling'.

Riedel, Rosenthal, Massanet and Lalique are four of the foremost producers in the world of beautiful glassware.

Advice from Voltaire

Voltaire, slender as a wand, wrote immortal prose. He himself lived to be a creditable, if not respectable, eighty-four. Perhaps his best advice, applicable to Slender Gourmets, was at the end of *Candide* when he reminded us to 'cultivate our garden'. Plant plenty of vegetables. Eat lots of green salads. Make sure that your salad bowl is as distinguished as your glassware and Champagne bucket. Choose a large roomy one, perhaps hand-carved out of an interestingly marked rich wood like olive. It should be spacious so that when you toss the contents each leaf is covered with a fine coat of dressing.

Moments of Madness

At the end of the meal you might indulge in a wild, wicked moment. Reach for the Laurent-Perrier bottle, turn it upside down, remove the cork from the opening in the butt, and release just one Champagne Truffle. These super chocolates are made at the Swiss Centre and come packaged in specially designed Champagne bottles. Sometimes the palate calls for a touch of sweetness to round off a perfect meal.

Pre-prepared Gourmet food – an Alternative to Cooking

If you don't want to cook, bring the products of one of the world's greatest Chefs into your own kitchen. 'Creative Cuisine' is a range of pre-prepared dishes planned by Michel Guérard and marketed by the chilled food specialists Chambourcy.

Michel Guérard, judging from recent photographs, is still slender, never having regained his former enormous girth. If he had I would not be recommending his new 'Creative Cuisine'. The proof of the pudding, in this case, is in the shape of the Chef.

This cuisine uses the freshest and best of raw materials; no preservatives, artificial colourings or flavourings are added. Sauces are prepared by blending wines, stock, herbs and a little cream, and reducing to a fraction of their original volume, thus getting a concentration of essential flavours and aromas.

Look for their range which includes Pork Medallions in Oriental Sauce and Chicken in White Wine and Tarragon in the chilled (not frozen) food department at Harrods and selected branches of Sainsbury.

6 *Following the Champagne Diet – Dining Out*

What Makes a Restaurant Great

The success of a restaurant depends on the policy of the Management, not to cut corners but to shop in the world markets daily and buy only the very best and freshest of ingredients.

The value of a Chef and staff is also of paramount importance as was appreciated only too well by the French aristocrats during the Revolution when they fled their country making sure that the most important members of their household escaped with them. Irrespective of their nearest and dearest it was often the Chef and the Sous Chef who escaped with the Marquis and settled in Soho where they opened restaurants.

Not only the ability but the philosophy of the Chef is vital to the success of a restaurant.

'If the Chef has not got the right attitude to cooking, the dish will be a failure – the soufflé will not rise.' So said Michael Quinn, ex-Chef of The Ritz.

It is important to visit restaurants that employ talented creative Chefs who mastermind the menus. Besides wanting to create great dishes, they must also be aware of food values, of health and diet, and who are open to new ideas and ways of cooking.

Traditional haute cuisine can be rich and heavy, sometimes providing a way for parsimonous cooks to save money by disguising inferior cuts of meat with thick, floury sauces. A lighter, simpler style of cooking is now favoured relying on the best ingredients which are enhanced (not disguised) with light sauces made by a reduction of mingled juices, wine and herbs. Lean cuts of meat are chosen, less butter and cream is used and subtler combinations of flavours, textures, aromas and colours are the rule, with a greater use of herbs and exotic fruits.

Pastry, puddings and flour-based dishes are kept to an absolute minimum and when served are in miniature sizes. The only pastry permitted is 'puff' – the air being calorie-free.

Again, as Michael Quinn said, 'A Chef cooks for the personal needs of the diner.' If the diner is an aspiring Slender Gourmet and not a fat glutton, then he will compose dishes with this image in mind.

Further, according to his philosophy, 'The cook must prepare food with love and care; otherwise, if he cooks carelessly, with indifference and a chip on the shoulder, then the dish will reflect his attitude.'

How often have you eaten out and been disappointed by the quality of the food? How often, for example, much to the distress of yourself and your guests, has the allegorical soufflé fallen flat on its face? To avoid this happening and to help you stay with your Diet I am listing some London restaurants that have my seal of approval.

The Calorie and The Count

It has been said that one's body is a Temple but we shouldn't devote ourselves only to prayer. Some luxuries, please. When in need of a calorie-cutting meal, visit one of these three Champagne, Caviar and Oyster bars where just one luxurious course costs only between 200 and 400 calories!

Otherwise, treat yourself and friends to a gastronomical experience at one of the other six restaurants listed in this Chapter. By judicious selection either on your part or on the Chef's, if you have a planned menu, you will still be able to leave the table feeling, and looking, like a Slender Gourmet.

Green's Champagne Bar. 36 Duke Street, St James's, S.W.1. – *London's 'buzziest'*

Green's Champagne Bar has the Gentleman's Club of St James's atmosphere with its dark panelled walls enlivened by Spy and Jak cartoons.

You can either sit in one of the mahogany dining alcoves if you want privacy, or you can watch the social whirl sitting at the semi-circular marble-topped bar. This is happily embellished with Champagne cooling in ice-buckets, accompanied by platters piled high with lobsters, crabs, oysters, langoustines and gulls' eggs.

A warm, friendly welcome awaits you from Mine Host, ex-guardee Simon Parker Bowles, Douglas, presiding in pin-striped trousers behind the bar, and Peter, who is probably the fastest oyster-opener in town, thirty oysters in seventeen seconds being his record.

Green's oysters come from the finest oyster beds in Poole and County Cork. The flavours are different; so experiment to see which you prefer. One can enjoy them with a drop of lemon, a couple of specks of cayenne pepper and, perhaps, a wafer-thin slice of brown bread and butter.

Don't attempt opening oysters yourself at home, prising the mollusc apart can lead to hand injuries and frayed tempers, and resorting to a hammer, chisel or pneumatic drill only gives the oyster a headache. Much better to leave it to an expert like Peter.

Follow the oysters with a plate of Green's smoked salmon, full of flavour, as it is caught swimming upstream, a hard excercise which makes it lean and low in fats. It has been smoked correctly, the old-fashioned way in brick holes over oak chippings. The method of smoking is all important to the final flavour.

Alternatively, you could choose Chef Beth Coventry's dressed Cornish crab and salad. It could as easily have come from Parnassus.

Oysters, salmon and crab, though simple fare, have complex mature flavours which cry out for a superb Champagne such as Laurent-Perrier's 'Grand Siècle', made from three great vintages. Cuvée No. 158 incorporates the vintages of 1966, 1969 and 1970. Described as 'the ultimate', 'the star in the crown', Simon Parker Bowles himself was moved to say that when his turbulent boat of life reaches quiet waters, he will rest in peace, provided he is accompanied with a few bottles of Grand Siècle, preferably Cuvée 158.

The Champagne Exchange, Curzon St., W.1. – *The Grand Unaffordables*

As caviar and the de luxe Champagnes are two of life's Grand Unaffordables, millionaires, and there are plenty of them around, should make them inseparable and free to their friends.

The first time I had those moist greyish eggs was in the Verandah Grill on the *Queen Mary*. A life-sized swan, carved out of glittering ice was trolleyed to my side, and there, buried deep in crushed ice, lay a stone pot containing a myriad of firm, plump Mallesol eggs.

On another occasion I was being entertained by a love-sick White Russian, who accompanied the Beluga eggs with songs sung in a sad, deep bass that turned to grief on presentation of the bill.

I haven't found either an iced swan or a love-sick Russian to embellish and dramatize the caviar presentation since, but in the restful, modern, pastel-toned interior of The Champagne Exchange, John Rushton will be delighted to meet you.

The Champagne Exchange has an extensive list of over fifty Champagnes which are sold by the glass, ½ bottle, bottle and magnum, ranging in quality from

Grandes Marques non-vintages to old vintages and Prestige Cuvées. Their policy is to serve delicacies that enhance their unique list of Champagnes.

Caviar is such a delicacy that it deserves the finest. A rare Champagne is the Dom Perignon 1966 at £145, with more recent vintages in a descending price scale, so that the Special Offer of Louis Roederer 1969 at £65 seems a gift.

Sitting comfortably at the Bar or at a table you can make your choice from three top caviars: Beluga, Osietra and Sevruga.

The Beluga eggs are the largest, generally grey in colour with a mild, creamy flavour.

The Osietra eggs are smaller with a slightly nutty taste.

The Sevruga eggs are the smallest and are generally black and tangy to the palate.

Living the Magical Moment

Whichever caviar you choose it will be served with chopped eggs and onions. Purists disapprove of these adornments because they disguise the delicate flavour of the roe. Toast points only are permitted; even a slice of lemon is suspect.

According to Mr Petrossian, owner of a well-known New York Caviar Bar, six or seven eggs should be trowelled directly on to the tongue from a gold-tipped palette (horn or bone will do), kept in the mouth for a second, then rolled on the tongue until the eggs burst against the palate, releasing their full flavour. Above all, he recommends that you don't talk or allow any external influences to detract your attention from the 'eggs-in-the-mouth moment'.

If you plan to eat caviar on a regular basis it might be as well to travel with your own palette as restaurants don't provide these ultra-refinements.

Reliving the Moment

When the eggs have disappeared, enjoy the after-taste. Open the mouth, let in a little oxygen which activates the latent aromas and flavour, then reach for your glass of Champagne.

How to Stretch your Caviar

A little caviar has to go a long way, as an average portion is twenty-five grams. One stretching method is to have it the popular way with buckwheat blinis and soured cream. Or alternatively in a jacket potato.

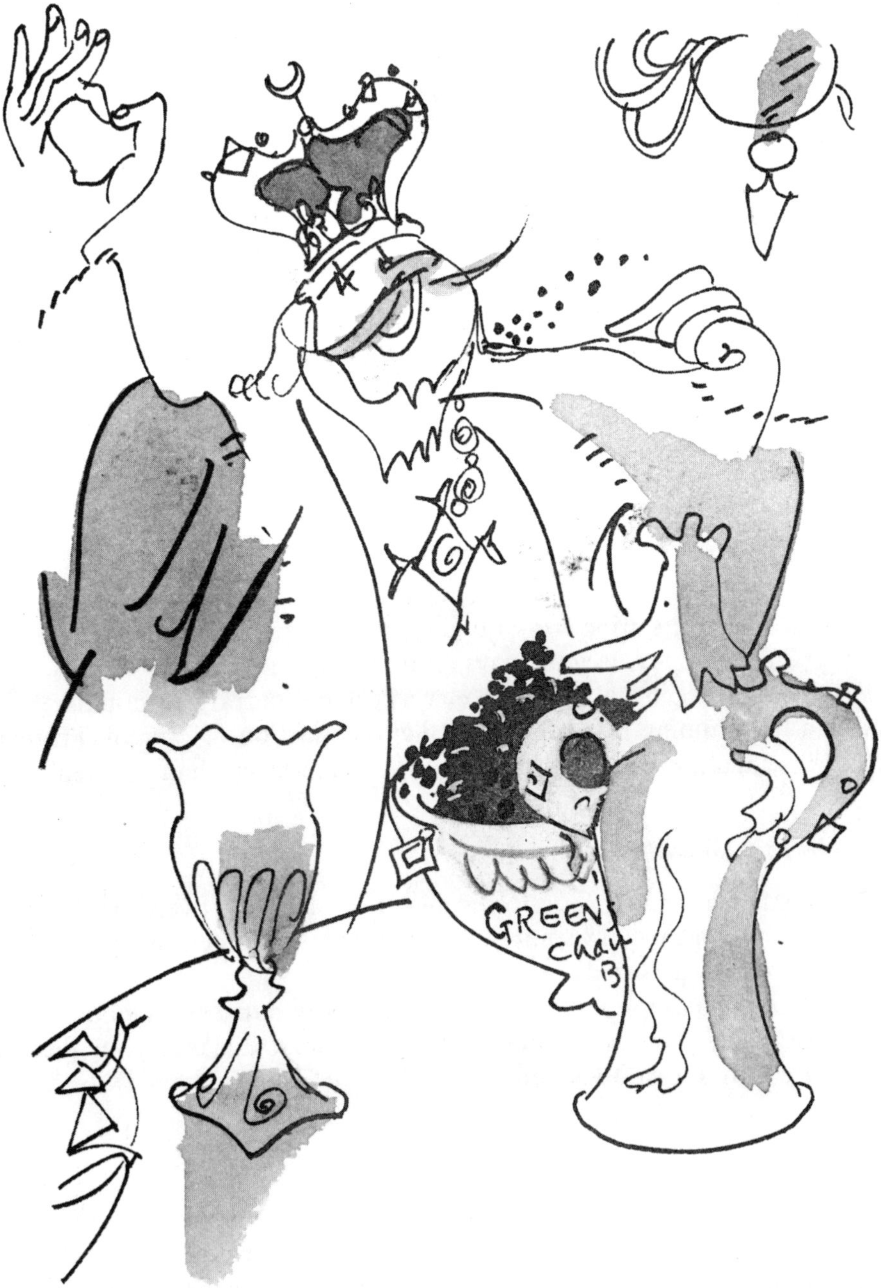

Caviar, to some people

Try the Slender Gourmet Stretch, twenty-five grams of caviar spread on a starter portion of smoked fish, which would be either salmon, sturgeon or halibut, accompanied by a green salad, two glasses of water and one of Champagne.

Scott's Restaurant, 20 Mount Street, W.1. – *The Divine Delectables*

Over the years Scott's has consistently enjoyed a reputation for being one of the best restaurants in London. Specializing in fish, whether it be Dover sole, turbot, halibut from Aberdeen, Cornish skate or Scottish salmon and lobster, it is always the best and it is deliciously prepared by Chef John Bertramo.

The Caviar Bar

Adjoining the restaurant, Scott's Caviar Bar has an air of elegant informality providing a perfect setting for enjoying an unhurried relaxed one-course meal.

On these calorie-conscious days you can pamper yourself with a Divine Delectable which can be, if you like, very rich. Contrary to popular belief rich food can be slimming if it contains a high proportion of protein. Protein clings to the ribs, making you feel that you have eaten more than you really have.

Divine Delectable No. I

This 200-calorie cutter is Les Royal Natives Nicholas, twelve selected oysters, gently poached in their own juices and covered with a delicate parmesan cheese sauce, before being glazed.

An oyster is a complete food containing all the nutrients the body needs and the cheese sauce provides a small amount of fat to balance your diet. Twelve oysters are only 60 calories and the cheese sauce approximately 120.

Divine Delectable No. II

If you like Champagne in your sauce as well as in your glass try the Cassolette d'Homard et St Jacques au Champagne, slices of lobster and scallops served with a delicate sauce of cream and Champagne. Believe it or not, this only comes to 210 for the lobster meat and 100 calories (two tablespoons of double cream) for the sauce. It has a rich extravagant flavour which makes dieting a pleasure.

Divine Delectable No. III

Caviar served with a small portion of steak tartar is an unusual taste combination. High in protein, you won't feel hungry for hours. With two slices of wholemeal toast this only comes to 400 calories allowing for a large serving of 100 grams of top Iranian caviar.

Watercress or a green vegetable would be an excellent accompaniment to any of these dishes.

Each of these meals allows you just one glass of the Slimmer's Champagne which is carbohydrate-free, either the Piper Heidsieck Sauvage or the Laurent-Perrier Brut. Your two glasses of mineral water are, of course, calorie-free.

Ninety Park Lane, W.1. –
Nights in the Gardens of West One

Everything about Ninety Park Lane is glamorous without being ostentatious, starting with the Hollywood-style canopied entrance that leads you from the bustle of Park Lane into the elegant grandeur of soft sofas, rich Renaissance colours and discreet antiques. Even a collection of portraits from Charles Forte's private art collection decorate the walls of the spacious dining room. The tables are arranged so that each one appears to command the best position in the room.

Truffle Festival Time

At various seasons throughout the year, countries, regions and their specialities are featured. During the truffle festival delicacies from Perigord highlight many of the dishes. Truffles will be found wrapped in slivers of chicken or appearing with sweetbreads and langoustine in light pastry cases. Another exoticism are balls of foie gras rolled in truffle dust or lettuce salad dressed with truffle juice.

Master-Minded by a Master Chef

Ninety Park Lane is fortunate in having its cuisine master-minded by Louis Outhier who runs one of France's 3 star Michelin-awarded restaurants in the South of France.

This great Chef received a classical training under the legendary Fernand Point of La Pyramide to which he has added his own interpretation of nouvelle and naturelle styles (low on saturated fats, sugar and artificial additives). His dishes are often flavoured with a hint of the East, spices, not the hot sort that set you on fire, but subtle, elegant aromas and flavours from Thailand.

Which Menu?

Should one choose from the à la carte or take a gastronomic adventure into the unknown with the Menu Surprise? I recommend the latter for Slender Gourmets with time on their hands to linger over eight courses, which will be relatively low on calories because the dishes are small, but each one a delight.

Oeuf Surprise

For a first course one might get some unusual eggs called Oeuf Surprise. Although at first glance these look like plain boiled eggs, albeit served in silver egg cups, they are, in fact, hot egg yolks with beluga caviar, surrounded by bitter cream, spiked with vodka to help the digestion. You need not feel guilty about the calories, the dish is small.

Hit the Highlights

Every meal must have its highlight; yours could be a brochette of langoustine and crayfish stuffed with lobster mousse and whole prawns served on a vegetable sauce accompanied by a dish of snow peas cooked with saffron stamens.

Or you might have the Truffles et St Jacques au Champagne, black truffles with white scallops in a Champagne sauce. Dishes composed in black and white remind me of the amusing story, which could only happen in France, of les Grandes Horizontales.

Les Grandes Horizontales

These ladies, known as les Grandes Horizontales, for obvious reasons, were mistresses of wealthy men. When the end of such an arrangement became necessary etiquette required that a *dejeuner de rupture* should take place. This gastronomic meal, every dish of which had to be composed in black and white, including the flowers and table decorations, was supposed diplomatically to convey the sad tidings. The lady's broken heart was more likely to be appeased if a little *cadeau* had thoughtfully been concealed in the petit fours. An alternative might be a jewel-encrusted Champagne bottle, its neck encircled with a dazzling diamond collar, such as the one recently designed by Van Cleef & Arpels to mark the bicentenary of Piper Heidsieck.

Perhaps the most surprising (or even dangerous) choice for a Slender Gourmet is the Caravanne des Desserts. A speciality of Ninety Park Lane, this multi-tiered

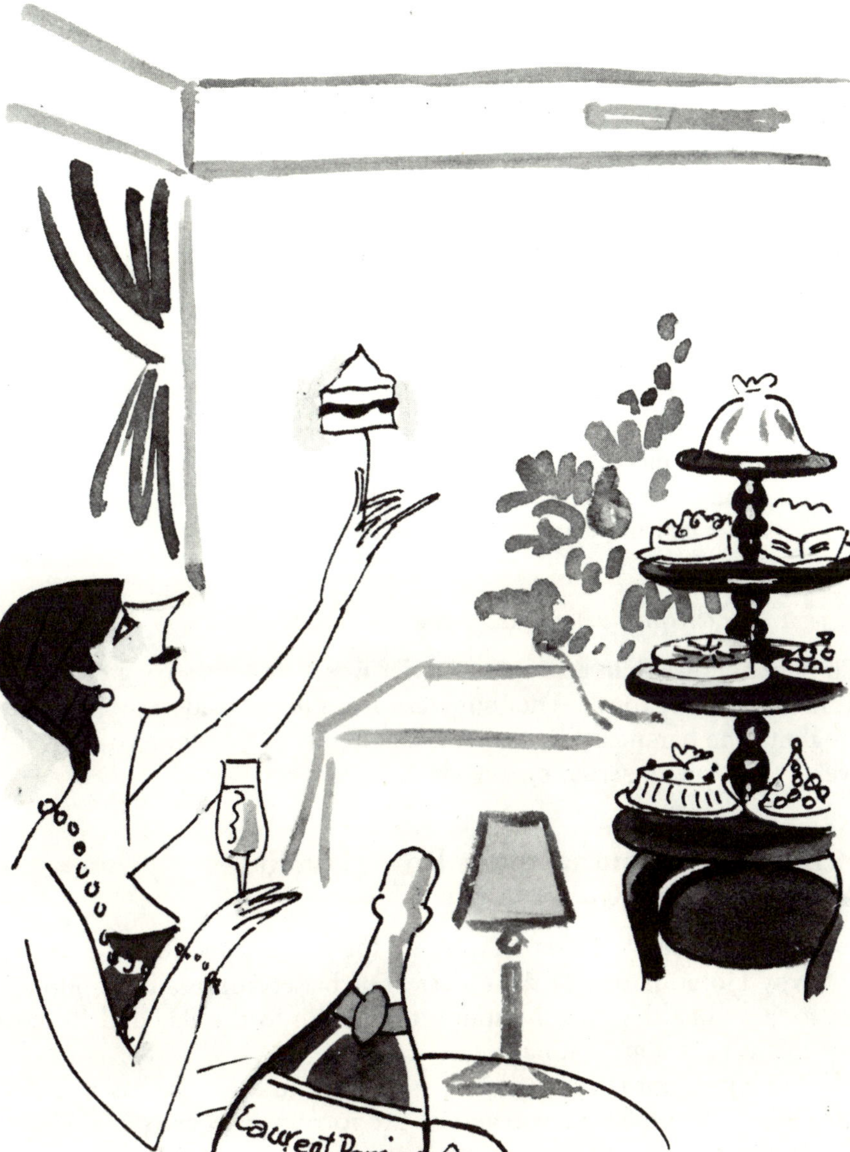

The Caravanne

pyramid on wheels looks like something out of 1001 Nights with its assortment of mousses, tarts, cakes, puddings and fruits, the loveliest sitting in shimmering splendour at the top.

Their desserts are exceptional. Artificial additives, food colours, flavourings and ersatz cream would never cross the kitchens of Ninety Park Lane. Only natural, fresh ingredients of the highest quality are used and the Slender Gourmet's downfall, sugar, is kept to the minimum.

Having said that, the Caravanne should definitely be counted in the major treat category – the lemon or pistache mousses being the least damaging to a Slender Gourmet's resolve with their delicate refreshing flavours. The more alcoholic mousses, raspberry with Eau de Framboises, orange with Grand Marnier or blackcurrant with Crême de Cassis, are invitations to disaster. Yet more devastating is the praline and hazelnut chocolate truffle cake.

However, the merest sliver, providing a taste sensation of one succulent mouthful, from your choice of three, would be permitted to the Slender Gourmet but not to the aspiring one.

To Accompany this Banquet

What better choice than a Laurent-Perrier Rosé, with its strong handsome colour and full fruity flavour? The bubbles are superb and will sing delightfully throughout the banquet and continue singing as they colour your cheek, leaving a lively, fresh tingly sensation on the palate.

Boulestin – Southampton Row, London –
A Temple to Gastronomy

Boulestin, in the heart of Covent Garden, theatreland and just over the road from The Savoy Hotel, is one of the oldest French Restaurants in London.

As soon as you descend the stairs that lead into the Bar and Restaurant you know this is a 'serious' eating place.

The Dining Room is comfortable, spacious and airy, yet has a cosy Clubland atmosphere. The tables have generous proportions and are positioned in a non-regimented way around the room. Pictures of cows and sheep munching in pastures look down on the tables of contented diners.

The cuisine is in the style of Escoffier, the great Chef of the Belle Epoque era, the forerunner of today's Nouvelle Cuisine, who said that sauces should be light and digestible and that vegetables are cooked 'al dente' to preserve their freshness and colour. Like Escoffier, Chef/Patron Kevin Kennedy is always searching for interesting ingredients and food combinations with an eye to colour, texture and flavour. Each dish is visually beautiful as well as succulently voluptuous. Also, like Escoffier, Kevin likes to keep his patrons fit and slim.

Fish is a feature. You might choose small parcels of salmon stuffed with foie gras, an escalope of salmon decorated with oysters in a marine and herb sauce, or, for the Champagne lover, a Coquilles Saint-Jacques au sabayon de Champagne.

Boulestin's menu follows the seasons and if you visit during *Printemps* the young Spring lamb en croute is a perfect choice. The purpose of the pastry is not to be eaten but to seal in all the delicious juices and aromas of lamb and herbs during cooking.

Slender Gourmets could indulge in occasional tastes but aspiring ones must be firm and leave all the pastry on the plate.

Vegetables are small, cooked *al dente* and both taste and look exquisite. I particularly like the celeriac served in crisp oval shapes substituting for the more prosaic, calorific mashed potato.

It takes two waiters to present the two heavily laden trays of French cheeses, but in view of their fat content, the merest sliver of two or three, selected for taste sensation only, is allowed the Aspiring Slender Gourmet. The Slender Gourmet can extend to four or five slivers.

A Champagne to accompany this repast might be the Perrier-Jouët Rosé, 'Blason de France' which is not found on many wine lists in England. It contains a high proportion of Chardonnay grapes from Perrier-Jouët's own premier vineyards in Cramant, and is divine.

'Tulipes' for dessert

Wafer thin bitter chocolate moulded into delicate tulip shapes act as edible containers for either raspberries and little strawberries or for a choice of sorbets. The smooth bitterness of the chocolate provides an excellent foil for both the soft fruits and sorbets. It's such a perfect taste combination that, in this instance, I would not leave anything on the plate. The Gourmet in you has to win sometimes.

The split-second timing of the service is perfect, the waiters are there the instant before you need them. They will also delightedly answer all your questions about the menu should Kevin be in the kitchens. You begin to feel that they love you if you love to eat. That, after all, is one of the great incentives to dining out.

Bracewell at the Park Lane Hotel, Picadilly – *Flambée Dining*

Bracewell's Restaurant in The Park Lane Hotel has been awarded a much coveted rosette for menu, service and ambience. The restaurant is plush in the Edwardian style, superbly carved oak panelling lines the walls which are highlighted by contrasting panels of ivory silk and bevelled glass – an elegant dignified dining room where Edward VII might have entertained Lillie Langtry. This tall squarish room is softened by circular tables, generous flower decorations, lots of silver, white linen and clear tulip-shaped glasses sparkling in the soft candlelight. Diners are ushered to their tables to the melodies of Cole Porter and Gershwin, played by pianist Perry Grant in the Cocktail Bar.

Chef Ian Whittock, trained in modern French cuisine, has perfected his five-course Menu Gastronomique, a combination of dishes that make the meal exceptional without being overly calorific, the portions are small but you are not left feeling hungry.

The Menu Gastronomique changes weekly. You might start with Milles Feuilles de Foie Gras au Cèpes, slivers of liver and mushrooms divided by wafer-thin pastry layers sitting on a hot creamy shallot sauce.

This could be followed by a light fish Soufflé using that Prince of fish, the Loup. The Soufflé surrounded by an orange flavoured sauce is ephemeral and delicate.

Then a water ice made from fresh raspberries which had been carefully rubbed through a sieve to remove the pips leaving the final Sorbet au Cassis as smooth as velvet.

For entree, perhaps Longe d'Agneau Mousseline a la Menthe, trimmed lamb cutlets bound with a mousseline of chicken flavoured with mint served on a rich port inspired sauce.

The vegetables can veer towards the unusual and imaginative such as Japanese Artichokes of which, I suggest, you form your own occidental opinion.

The dessert looked marvellous, a biscuit base filled with peach, apricot and icecream topped with gossamer fine layers of silvery spun sugar. This sugary hat is removable, one small nibble only being permitted.

We forego this Timbale Amelia in favour of the Crêpes.

Crêpes Suzette – Flambée!

Few restaurants cook at your table, douse the food with alcohol and set it alight. This is partly for fear of scorching the walls or setting off the fire alarm, which activates the ceiling sprinklers, which in turn would drench the diners.

When Restaurant Manager Oscar Bassam is a Fellow of the Acadamie

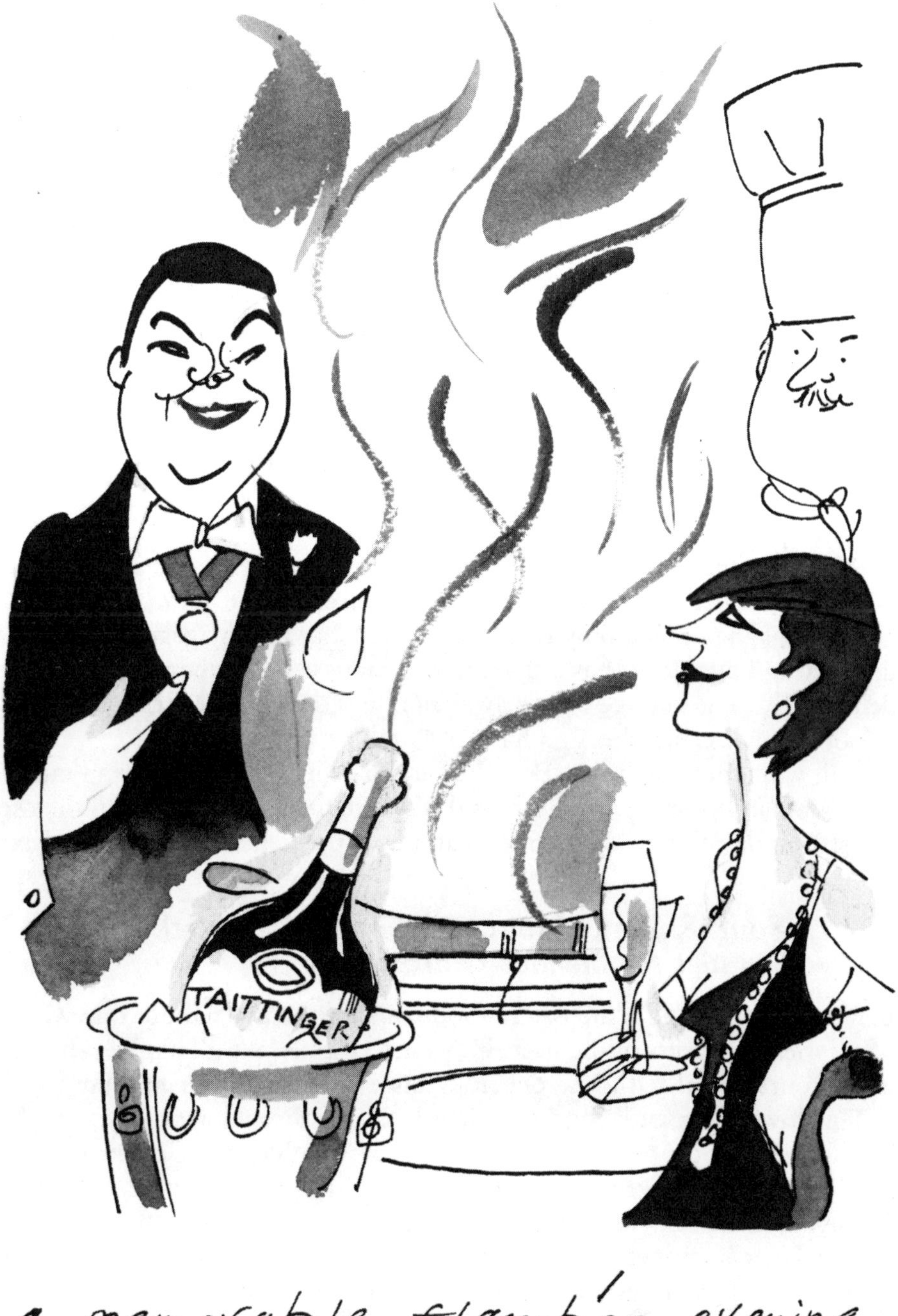

a memorable flambée evening

Internationale de Flambier and has won worldwide awards, it would be a tragedy if the meal didn't, at some course, go up in flames.

Mr Oscar, immaculately dressed, carnation in buttonhole, presides behind the flambée trolley on which stands the crêpe mixture, freshly squeezed oranges and lemons and bottles of Grand Marnier, Curaçao and Brandy.

He peels a whole orange and spears the thick length of skin on to a long rapier handed him by the Chef. Holding it high over the skillet of bubbling crêpes, he pours an ignited ladle of brandy slowly down the spiralling peel so that the burnt zest drips into the crêpes along with the brandy. Flames leap ceilingwards to the delight of the diners. You almost feel like applauding such superb showmanship.

In case the Crêpes sound overindulgent, do remember a gourmet's allegiance is to fine food and if it's a little over the calorific odds, don't worry, there is the 'morning after 30 calorie breakfast' to adjust the balance.

Bracewell's Restaurant benefits from an excellent wine cellar built up over the years by the family who own the hotel. Their Fine Wine Club allows members a 25% discount which almost makes a bottle of Champagne an economical buy.

Taittinger's Champagnes are well represented on the Wine List. Their 'Comtes de Champagne', made only from the white Chardonnay grape, is the ultimate in delicacy and quality. It has a fine rarified mousse and, when held to the ear, sings delightfully. The vintage currently available is the '79, but Bracewell's have a rare '75 on their list and the '75s have a 4-star rating.

Following the rules of the Diet, be sure to order a bottle of Evian mineral water to accompany your wine. This brand is one that is light and soft, unlike some that are strong on mineral salts which can mask the delicate flavour of Champagne.

Le Soufflé, Hotel Intercontinental, Hyde Park Corner, W.1. – *A Banquet for Slender Gourmets*

Banquets on a grand scale where food consumed equals about one week's supply of calories are events of the past. However, at times we all hanker after a splendid multi-course meal with one delicious taste sensation after another.

This love affair with food can play havoc with your waistline, but Le Soufflé has solved this problem with their Banquet for Slender Gourmets' offering the Chef's choice of seven courses. Each dish is small, low in calories, high in nutrients, and looks and tastes exquisite.

Chef Peter Kromberg changes his menu every three or four days, planning each menu around the finest, freshest ingredients available.

An Evening's Entertainment

Decorated in Art Deco style, the restaurant provides a spacious, comfortable setting for your feast. Indulge, but don't rush, otherwise you'll get indigestion. Allow a few hours to bask in delicious food, Champagne, perfect service and your companion(s).

That evening Chef Kromberg presented us with a tartar of salmon topped with sour cream and flecked with chives. One of the best ways to cook certain fish is by marinating in a light oil and lemon juice. For this particular dish Chef Kromberg selected wild salmon in preference to its pool-farmed brother because it has a leaner, firmer texture. Non-fatty fish and meat, of course, are what keep Gourmets slender.

This was followed with a feuillette of morilles fraiches, black wrinkled mushrooms that have a delicate yet distinctive, slightly aromatic flavour. They look ugly but taste heavenly.

Then a petit marée of fishes selected for contrasting texture and flavour, individual 1 oz. circles of langoustine, scallops, lobster, red mullet and John Dory, steamed separately so that flavours don't overlap, served sitting on a vegetable sauce garnished with red and black caviar eggs. One of the purest ways of cooking fish is by steaming because it retains all the goodness and flavour.

The mid-Banquet sorbet was made from blackcurrants, crème de cassis and a Mercury wine from Beaujolais.

To complement the multiplicity of dishes, a pink Champagne with serious overtones, like the Louis Roederer Rosé, would be a perfect choice.

That evening the *piece de résistance* was filets of beef served with foie gras and truffles. Filet, unlike rump or sirloin steak, is low in fat and can be relied upon to be tender. The sauce, thickened by a natural reduction of juices, is non-fattening, as are all Chef Kromberg's sauces.

Cheeses appeared with a complement of luscious black grapes providing enzymes that help metabolize fats.

A '*nouvelle-esque*' finale to the meal was poached pears sliced into a fan pattern sitting on a red sauce made from a purée of fresh passion fruit (not the canned variety), providing the natural sweetness to maintain the sugar level in the blood.

This is a 'banquet' for those who want to eat the finest, freshest food, a cuisine that satisfies the soul and nourishes the body.

The Four Seasons – Inn on the Park Hotel, Park Lane – *Dine Gourmet-Style on 750 calories*

A 750-calorie dinner at the Four Seasons Restaurant in the 5-star Inn on the Park Hotel sounds improbable. Visions of undressed lettuce leaves, crudities and plain grills flashed through the mind, the sort of food that is definitely slimming but oh, so boring.

As it happened, a recent visit turned into something of an experiment in calorie-counting.

Entering the elegant restaurant we felt that austerity surely couldn't exist in such sumptuous surroundings. Sinking into the depths of a softly cushioned banquette I began to feel very hungry, so persuaded my friend to try the diplomatically described 'alternative cuisine' – the 750-calorie menu, which was low in fats and salt, while I would revel in the à la carte.

At the outset he rejected asparagus with fresh herbs, choosing instead, Lobster salad with mango, whilst I planned to live it up on Lobster Royale, a half baby lobster mousse garnished with caviar, tomato and basil dressing. He too had a half baby lobster served with a finely shredded salad of escarole, radicchio, chicory and mango, topped with a soupçon of dressing, achieving a finesse of flavours which my richer counterpart lacked.

To follow, he chose French pigeon, cooked in its own juices which had been reduced and flavoured with port. This was accompanied by a Timbale of carrots, mange tout and celeriac.

My choice was the Filet of Veal flamed with armagnac, served with a cream sauce and morille mushrooms. Two filets of veal represent about half a pound of meat, which is too much protein, especially with a heavy sauce. His 5 oz. portion of protein was the right size, succulent to the taste, and the slightly sweet sauce, though light, stood up to and counteracted the richness of the bird. Again I preferred his entrée to mine.

My guest concluded his meal with a combination of fresh fruits in a coulis of strawberries, whilst impulsively I chose a Crême Brulée with its crunchy caramelized top covering a rich cream filling. A Slender Gourmet's downfall – 576 calories – charged with cholesterol.

Being let loose on the à la carte is dangerous; much wiser to keep to the carefully monitored menu, especially when it is so good.

He thought that a light, frothy Champagne would marry well with his 750 calories, so we chose the bottle with the distinctive red sash of merit across the front, the Mumm Cordon Rouge. Intermingled, but not in the glass, with a lightly mineralized Volvic Water.

This calorie-controlled 'Alternative Cuisine' is presented by Chefs Eric Deblonde and Philippe Boulet and is perfect for the Aspiring Slender Gourmet and for those who have, for medical reasons, to watch all manner of biological facts of life.

If you are jet-setting around the big cities in America, Canada and England, visit the restaurants in the Four Seasons Group; they all present this 'Alternative Cuisine' and for those who are really thinking thin there is a 600-calorie menu as well.

Maxim's, Leicester Square, W.C.1. – *Dance the Night (and calories) Away*

Shakespeare was inspired to write in his Seven Ages of Man of 'seeking the bubble reputation in the cannon's mouth'. Better to find it at Maxim's.

You no longer need travel to Paris to visit this legendary restaurant. You need only go as far as London's Leicester Square where it has been faithfully reproduced down to the smallest detail. The same spacious bar and restaurant layout, wall mirrors ensconsed with golden scrolly curves, subdued lighting that makes everyone look beautiful – it is all here. One even has a feeling that Toulouse-Lautrec or Sarah Bernhardt might appear at any moment.

Ever since Franz Lehar immortalized Maxim's de Paris in his operetta *The Merry Widow*, the name has become synonomous with the world of diplomats and barons, beautiful actresses and wealthy widows; where Champagne flowed, diamonds sparkled, food was of the finest and a plethora of gypsy violinists played the night away.

London's Maxim's like its Parisian counterpart, has glamour and attracts a clientelle from the theatre and associated arts as well as captains of industry and jet-setting entrepreneurs.

The gypsy violinists are no more, but a small ensemble plays music to dine to, increasing in volume and tempo as the evening progresses and the diners take to the floor.

Instead of the prosaic three-course Club Menu choose a classical French dish from the à la carte. This might be rich but dancing between courses will consume some of the calories.

Typical dishes are Bouillabaisse à la Parisienne – sole, red mullet, scampi, mussels and whiting simmering in a saffron, tomato, garlic and leek sauce, served with crunchy fried croutons. (The croutons to be crunched by Slender Gourmet's only). Or, Navarin de Fruits de Mers Sous Cloches – sole, turbot, scallops, langoustines and sea bass tossed in a white wine and cream sauce and served *sous cloches*, under a glass bell. When the bell is removed the aromas are released, enhancing the overall enjoyment of the dish.

Either of the above could be preceded by a salad and followed by a fruit-based dessert.

The IN Champagne at Maxim's de Paris at the turn of the century was Perrier-Jouët's Belle Epoque which comes in the beautiful flower-decorated bottle. So, what better choice than a bottle of this nectar to put you into the truly gay mood of Maxim's?

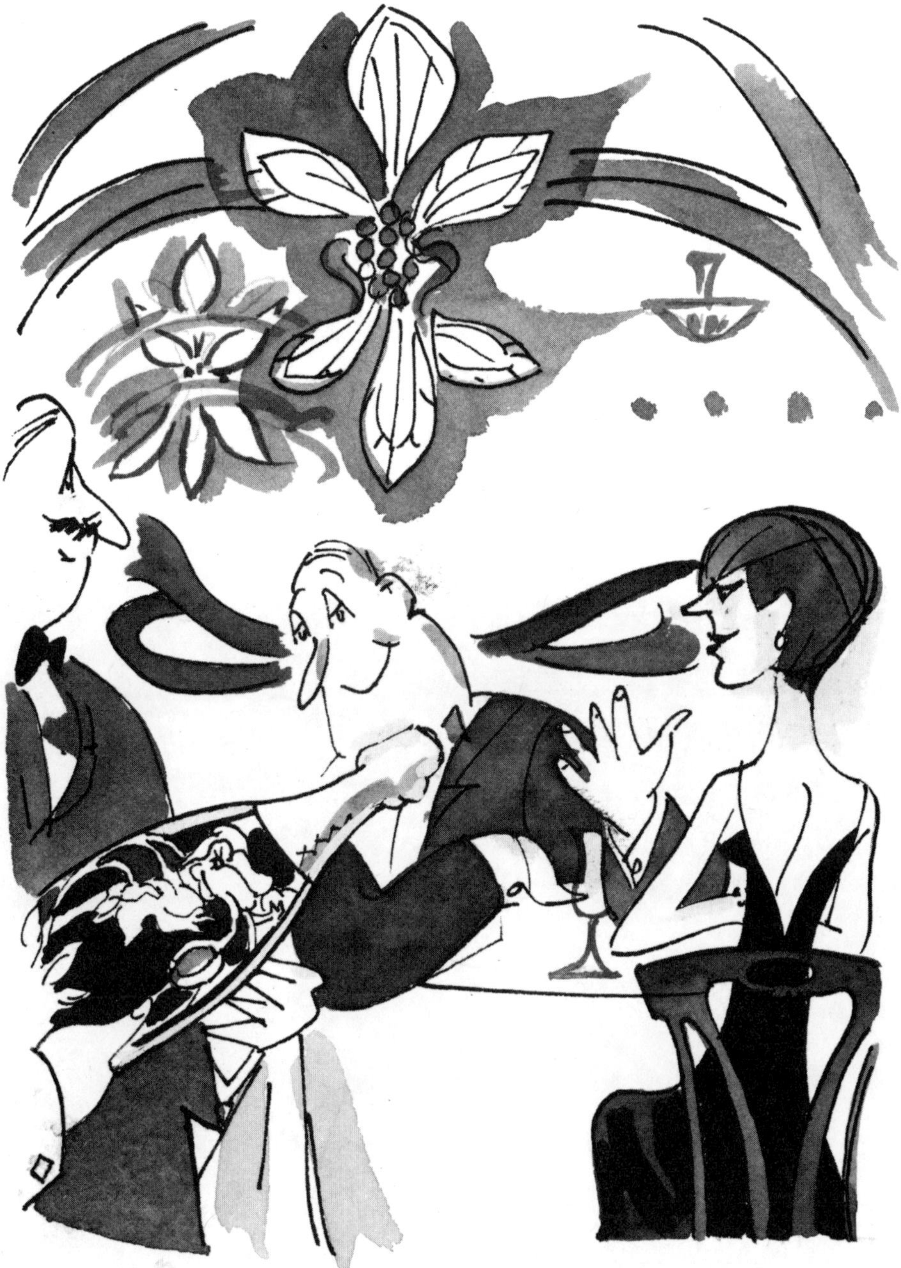

maxim's

7 *Take A Deep Breath*

The problem with many sporting activities is that one has to be fit in order to 'keep fit' playing them.

Tennis and squash fall into this category. Golf and bowls are less energetic, but they barely reach the stomach muscles; rowing develops the chest, arms and shoulders and cycling enhances the calves.

Although these sports will tone you up most effectively, there are other gentler activities that should not be overlooked such as dancing, deep breathing and incidental exercise. For the more adventurous, as already suggested, why not try a trip in a hot air balloon or take up sailing?

Dancing

Disco has certain advantages over ballroom, a partner being superfluous, you can make your movements as energetic or casually elegant as you choose.

A good movement for Aspiring Slender Gourmets is the Hip Twist Step that works the hips and waist in all the right directions.

Hip Twist Step

Stand with your feet about a foot apart, toes facing front.
Point the ball of your right foot outwards to 3 o'clock.
Then turn the right foot inwards to face 9 o'clock.
Repeat eight times with the right foot, eight times with the left foot.
There are lots of variations you can develop from this one basic step.

Whether you are dancing at Maxim's or on your own at home, play your favourite piece of music whether it be disco, jazz, rock, soul or country, as long as it's got a good rhythmical beat that makes you want to move.

Give yourself space and *flow* . . .

Start with the shoulders, making half circles back and forwards; then stretch the neck, cat-fashion, from side to side. Shake your arms and hands, give at the knees and finish off with the Hip Twist Step above. God bless America!

Breathe the Years and Pounds Away

Correct breathing is a pleasurable, non-exhausting activity especially when the air is fresh.

Air contains oxygen and we need oxygen to feed and cleanse the blood. This, in turn, travels throughout the body, revitalizing and nourishing every muscle, ligament, cellular tissue, organ, nerve and gland.

Deep breathing exercises the lungs, ribcage and the auxilliary muscles attached to the abdomen. These in turn massage the internal organs, helping the digestion and assimilation of food.

Yogis, who have worked out a complete health and exercise system based on deep-breathing techniques, believe that 'the more and deeper you breathe the younger you get'. If you can honestly say that you breathed deeper and better quality air the preceeding year why become a year older when you feel a year younger?

By following the Champagne Diet and breathing deeply you will be able physically to deduct a year (or two or three) next birthday.

A fact that people don't realize and what every Aspiring Slender Gourmet should know is that, apart from the years, the POUNDS can also be breathed away! The theory is that the process of metabolism is speeded up by an extra intake of oxygen.

Breathing Exercise No. 1. The Deep Breath, which benefits all parts.

BREATHE IN slowly and deeply, being aware of the ribcage expanding sideways as the lungs fill with life-giving oxygenated air.

BREATHE OUT just as slowly and deeply, being aware of the ribcage falling inwards as the old, polluted carbon dioxide leaves the body.

Breathing Exercise No. 2. The Dog Pant.

BREATHE quickly, IN and OUT, through the mouth (as though you have been running and are out of breath).

Combine this with quick, small tummy pulls, in and out.

Breathing Exercise No. 3. The Sitali Breath.

Place tongue between the lips so that just the tip protrudes.

BREATHE IN slowly through the mouth. Withdraw the tongue and close the lips.

BREATHE OUT slowly through the nostrils.

When proficient, add a stomach retraction.

At the end of BREATHING OUT withdraw the stomach inwards, towards the spine.

Incidental Exercising

These are exercises that can be done during the course of your daily round of activities, like walking short distances rather than using the car, using stairs instead of the lift and walking the escalators rather than riding them.

In Japan it is not unusual for businessmen and women to break into a two minute exercise session, sometimes on the hour, every hour, during the day.

At the sound of a bell everyone stops talking, stands up, bows politely to each other and goes through a few stretch and twist movements before resuming where they left off.

Small doses of frequent exercise are more effective than strenuous longer sessions tackled once a week. Simple tummy 'pull ins' with short 'hold' periods, for example, can be done whilst shaving, under the shower, having a bath, travelling, sitting at the desk, on the phone and in bed.

All these little two-three minute exercise breaks add up to double figures by the end of the day.

Speed up your Metabolism

One of my favourite spots for breathing fresh clean air, far away from polluted city streets and traffic fumes, is in a hot air balloon. Why not glide up, in a beautiful balloon, to the rarefied atmosphere of a thousand or so feet? Drifting lazily over hills, trees, meadows and lakes, the air sparkles with a crisp, fragrant freshness like that of a good Champagne. Take in lots of deep breaths and say to yourself 'I am breathing the POUNDS away'.

Hot air ballooning attracts a large number of enthusiasts who traditionally arrive with lots of bubbly.

In the old days three or four people would clamber into the basket taking the Champagne with them and use the bottles as ballast. After drinking the contents they would discard them to gain height (which is unkind to those on the ground whose property or person could get hit by falling glass).

These days most hot air ballon excursions are divided into two parties; those who go up in the balloon and those who follow the balloon's progress in a Champagne-filled Landrover.

When the balloon descends, often into a favoured flowerbed or, worse still, a field of nurturing crops, the wrath of the property owners has to be appeased somehow. At this point, the Landrover arrives, the butler jumps out and starts pulling the corks, a multi-explosion of pops, the balloonists, Landrover squad, horticulturalists and farmers are soon united in the joys of an impromptu Champagne party.

A less exhilarating alternative to ballooning is to sit under a tree. Trees give off oxygen and obligingly take in the carbon dioxide that we breathe out, which is a convenient two-way exercise for both the breather and the tree.

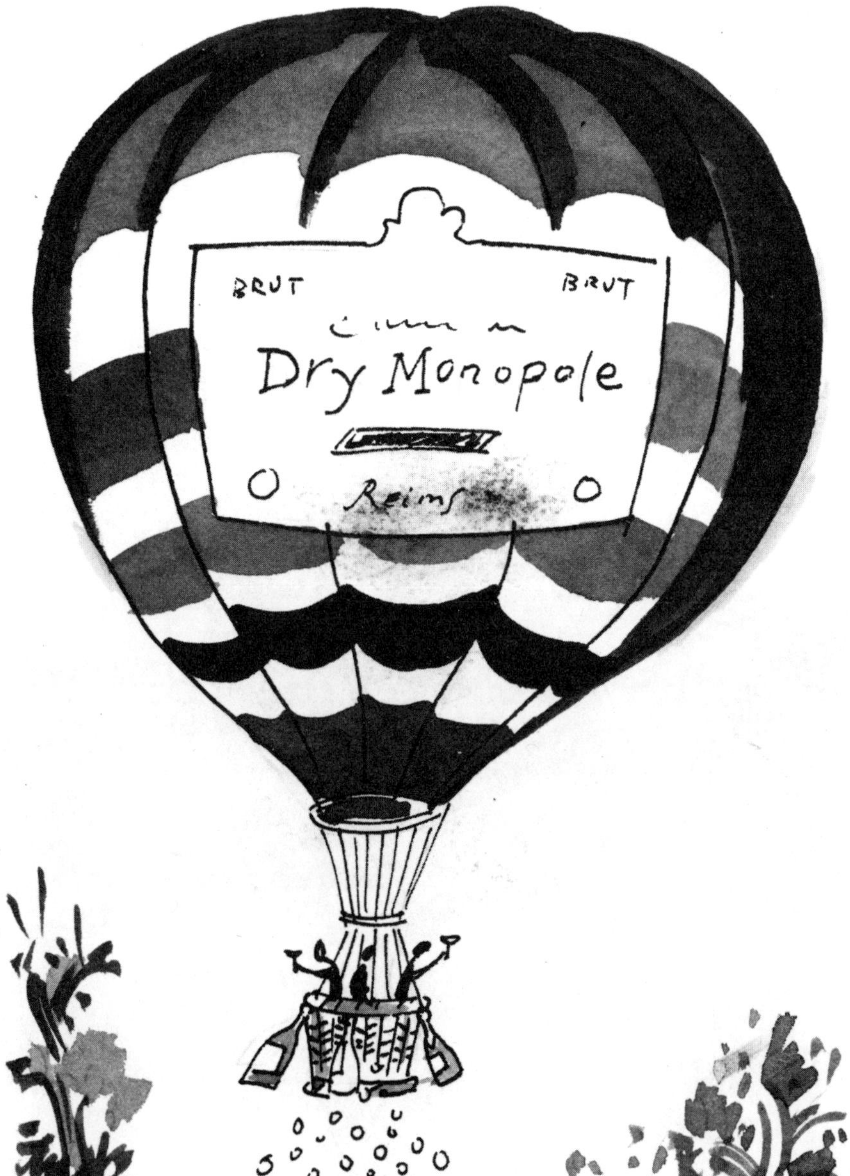

the rarefied atmosphere

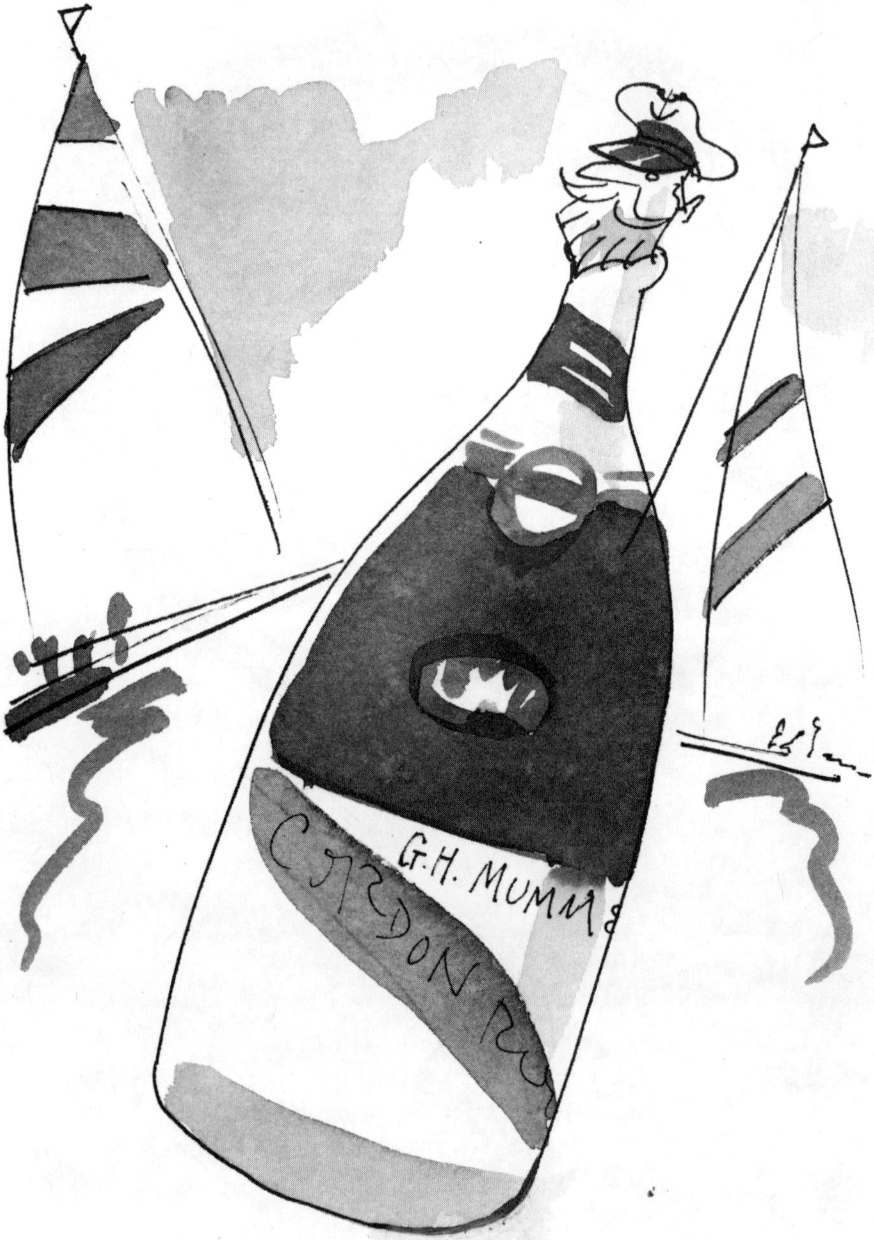

the winning skipper

Yachting is so Bracing . . .

Whether you be sitting on the side of a sailing dingy, feet braced against the gunnel, or standing on a wind-surfing board, the body acting as counter-balance to the wind and sails keeps the stomach muscles flexed ready for action, such as falling overboard, clambering back into the boat is excellent exercise.

By the way, if you are a yachting enthusiast and took part in one of the famous races such as the Admiral's Cup, which is sponsored by Mumm's Cordon Rouge Champagne, you could win your weight in bubbly! You'll also get the cheers and applause of the multitude which is good for the psyche. Think of it, thirteen or fourteen stone converted into bottles and magnums, even Jeroboams!

Champneys Health Club, Meridien Hotel, Picadilly

It is a good idea to join a Health Club. One of the most luxurious in London is Champneys whose facilities include squash courts, a swimming pool complete with marbled nymphs, a fern-graced jacuzzi and a gym equipped with the latest exercise machines.

After your fitness assessment test you could give yourself a leisurely workout and relaxation session, don a comfortable track suit and initiate yourself into exercise by 'spot-pacing' on the electronic treadmill? This moving carpet strip is monitored by a self-operated timer allowing you to decide whether to take a walk, trot, jog or break into a run.

Jogging, or any aerobic activity, strengthens the heart muscle and helps reduce the heart-attack risk, which means you have more years ahead in which to follow the Champagne life-style.

The Sit-Up Board, in the gym, is good for toning up and strengthening the stomach muscles. It's very popular as it allows you to be in a recumbent position, with your legs and hips raised half of the time. The other half is spent executing a series of sit-ups.

Oh, hang it all . . .

Hanging by the hands or feet, provided it's not the neck, is very good for you; it stretches the spine and gives the body that elegant, elongated El Greco look (as opposed to a Rubens cherub). An alternative to free-style hanging is a vertical board which clasps your body and can be adjusted to the angle of your choice. A couple of seconds, or minutes, with your head pointing to Australia is both physically and mentally stimulating, which is why some people do their best thinking standing on their heads.

Don't overdo the exercise; beginners should take it easily, interspersing physical activity with bouts of stretching and relaxing. Eventually you can join the more proficient and give your muscles something of a challenge.

The Aspiring Slender Gourmet should now have a swim around the Grecian marbled goddesses in the blue-mosaic-tiled pool. Twelve metres of warm blue water provide the space for an acquatic workout and when set in surroundings of cool, neoclassical splendour makes one feel either like a Roman Emperor or Venus rising from the sea.

Stepping into the jacuzzi is by contrast, hot and peaceful, the only sound coming from jets of water releasing a steady stream of pulsating bubbles that caress and massage the shoulders and back, leading perhaps to thoughts of other bubbles that sing in the glass.

Facts about Abdominals

The old portraits of handsome generals surveying the scene of battle, with broad shoulders, neat waistlines and diminishing hips, often depended on a tightly laced corset to hold everything in. Nobody needs go to those uncomfortable lengths today, provided that they keep their own built-in muscular corset fully toned-up. Nature's corset is designed to hold the abdomen and its contents firmly in place for a lifetime of wear.

Your Corset

The abdominal corset is made up of muscles that go diagonally, horizontally and vertically over the stomach area. The upper part is flanked by the ribcage and the lower half by the pelvic bones. This muscular corset holds in not only the flesh but the abdominal contents as well. Think of it – fifty metres of intestine as well as heavy organs like the stomach, liver, bladder, pancreas and spleen. If this muscular corset slackens these contents can fall out of alignment, pushing against

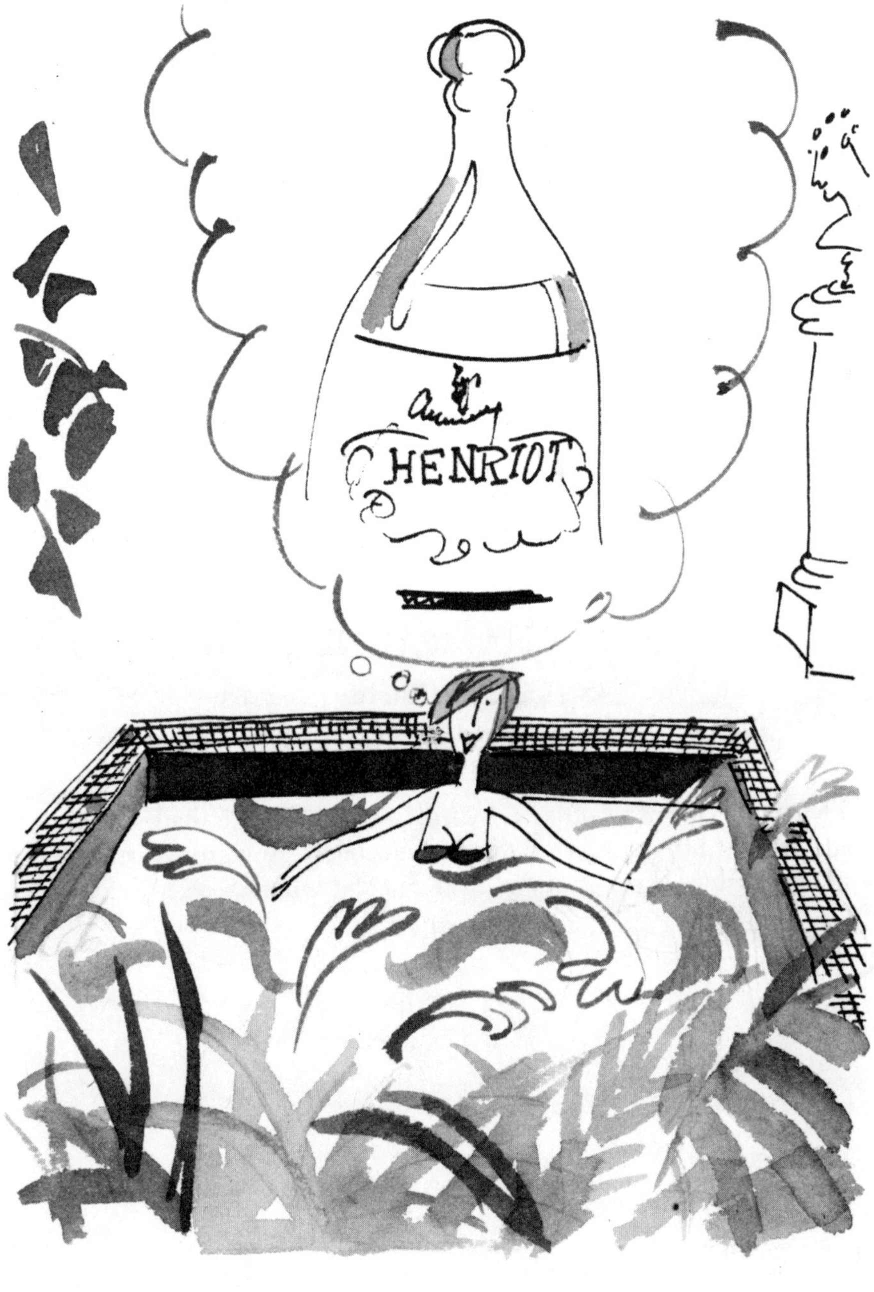

Jacuzzi

the abomindal wall, making a protuberance; but, worse still, if these organs are squashed together minor and major health disorders develop, ranging from ulcers to severe cases of indigestion affecting the heart, pulmonary veins and arteries.

According to an article in the *British Medical Journal* people with *largesse* are regarded as high heart-attack and stroke risks. For health, fitness and appearance the stomach muscles are the most important ones to keep in first class condition.

Why, you may ask, do those surplus pounds always settle around the middle rather than build up on the legs, arms, chest or hips? It's because the abdomen, that fleshy area extending from the ribcage to the pelvic girdle is the part of the body that gets exercised the least.

You need special exercises to tone-up and strengthen the abdominals and that's why you should try and spend five to ten minutes every morning, and evening, doing the CHAMPAGNE QUARTET.

There is no need to suffer the discomfort of a chilly floor; instead, why not do them in the comfort and warmth of your bed? Exercising in bed is part of the Champagne luxury image.

THE CHAMPAGNE QUARTET

'Champagne Charlie is my name,
Champagne Drinking is my game . . .
The Champagne Quartet is my aim . . .'

The singer of this popular Edwardian Music Hall ballad would certainly have tried, provided there was sufficient inducement. Reward yourself with a bottle of your favourite when you have mastered the Quartet.

The exercises consists of: Half Sit-Ups
Waist Turns
Full Sit-Ups
The Champagne Challenge

Half Sit-ups

Works lower abdominals

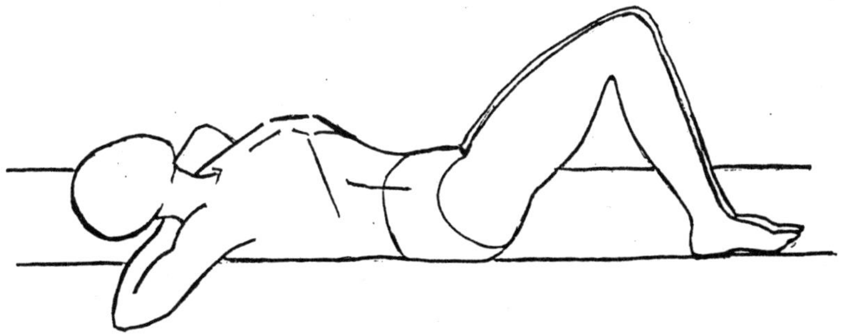

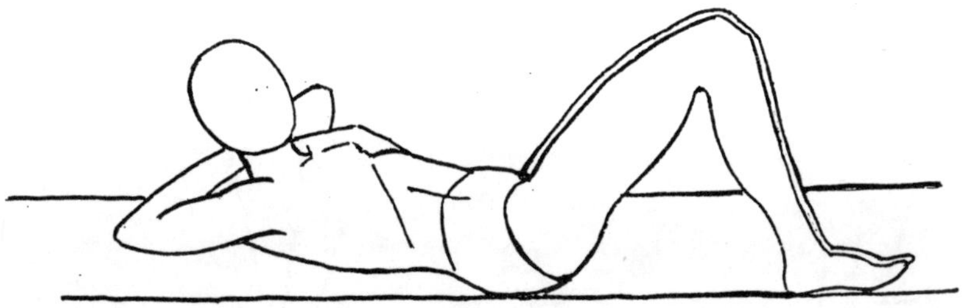

Push aside the pillows so that your head lies flat on the mattress. Link fingers, hands behind neck, elbows back. Bend knees, feet flat.

Lift your head and upper back, keeping your elbows parallel to the mattress. Lower body.

Start by doing 8 Slow – Pause, 12 Quick – Rest.

Increase the number of rounds when your stomach muscles say 'yes'.

WAIST TURNS

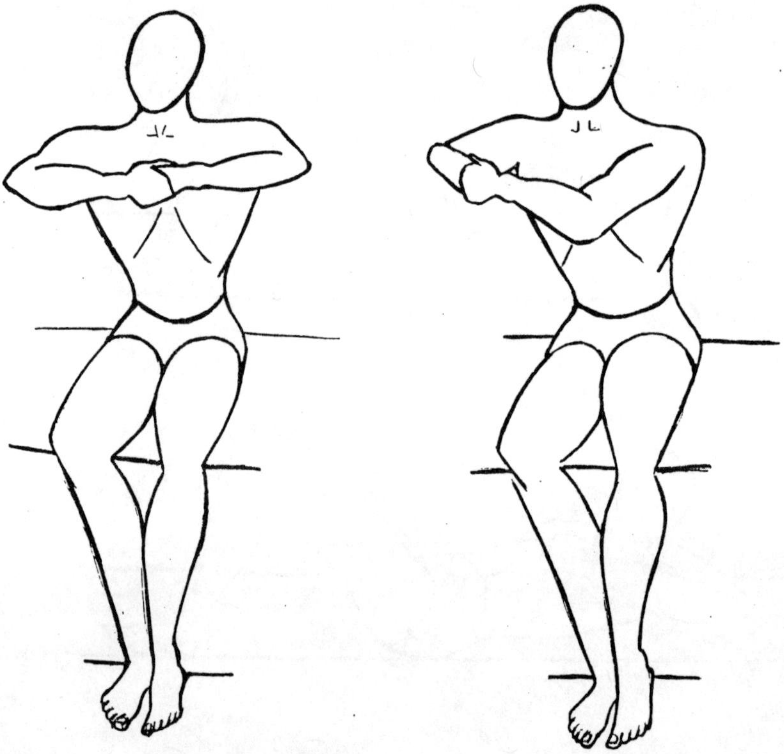

Sit on the edge of the bed for these turns and also for the Full Sit-Ups that follow.

Face front, arms folded, hold away from the body at chest level.

8 turns to the Right
8 turns to the Left
Then 6 each side, 4 and finally 2.

FULL SIT-UPS

Works lower and upper abdominals

The Easy Way – Easy because you can grip the edge of the bed with the back of your thighs and knees. This helps enormously.

Lie flat, arms overhead, swing up to a sitting position, bend forward, sit up, round back, lie down.

Try 6 to start with then gradually increase the number of repetitions each week.

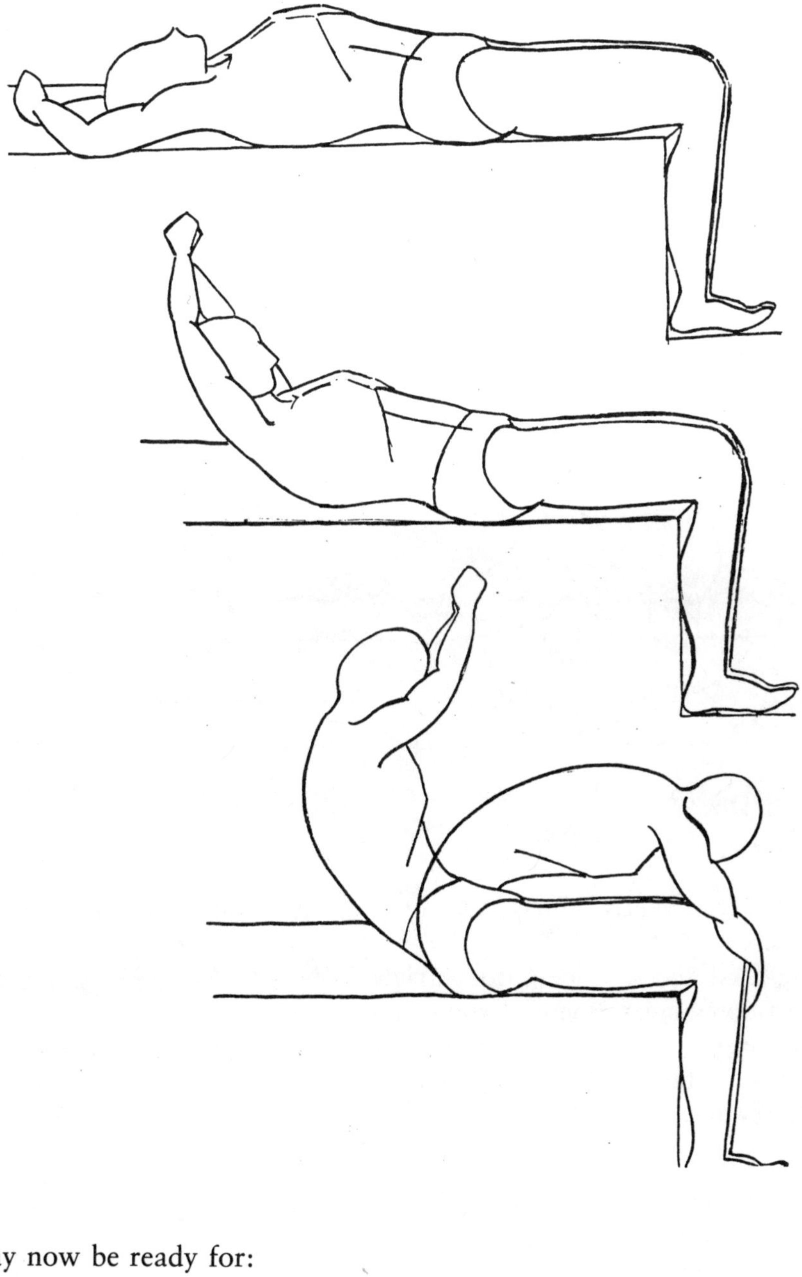

You may now be ready for:

The Champagne Challenge

Works all the stomach muscles, up, down across and verticals.
The 'Challenge' is hard, so save it until the other three become relatively easy.

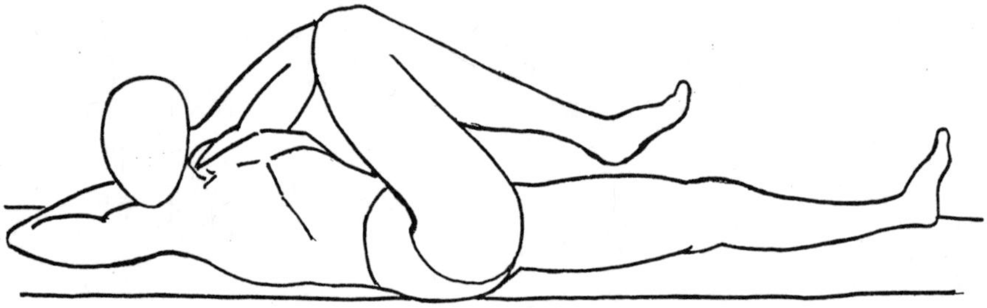

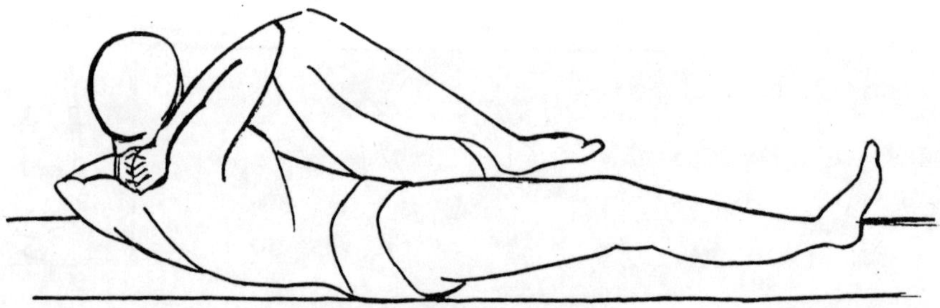

Lie flat. Clasp hands behind head, keep one leg straight the other knee bent in to the chest.

Lifting head and shoulders, touch right knee with left elbow and vice-versa.

Start by doing one round of 8, pause and ask yourself how you feel. Depending on the answer, you will get an idea as to how many rounds your body can do.

Set yourself a target – four, six, eight or ten rounds and when you succeed reach for your reward.

Champagne Posture

Whether you are standing, walking, sitting behind a desk or on a stool in your favourite Champagne bar, develop a relaxed yet alert posture.

Resist the downward pull of gravity by stretching upwards through the crown of the head. Make sure that your shoulders are relaxed.

Thinking tall makes you pull inwards from the waistband which immediately takes a couple of inches off the waist and stomach.

Good posture also injects your personality with a bon viveur sparkle and projects confidence and good health.

The Dangerous Plateau

You followed the Champagne Diet for a week or two, the scales indicated a weight loss of between two and five pounds, and then disaster struck, the scales would not budge.

Don't become discouraged and throw in the Champagne; you have hit the customary Dangerous Plateau, a period when the pounds will not diminish.

Take heart, the pounds may not be moving but the waistline inches are. The initial weight loss is mainly water and exercises build up muscle which weighs more than flesh; you may weigh the same but your shape will be firmer and slimmer.

Think Champagne Posture, pull away from your waistline and you may find you can tighten your belt by an extra notch.

This Dangerous Plateau period will pass within a couple of weeks, especially if you eat a little less and exercise a little more, you will resume your encouraging weight loss.

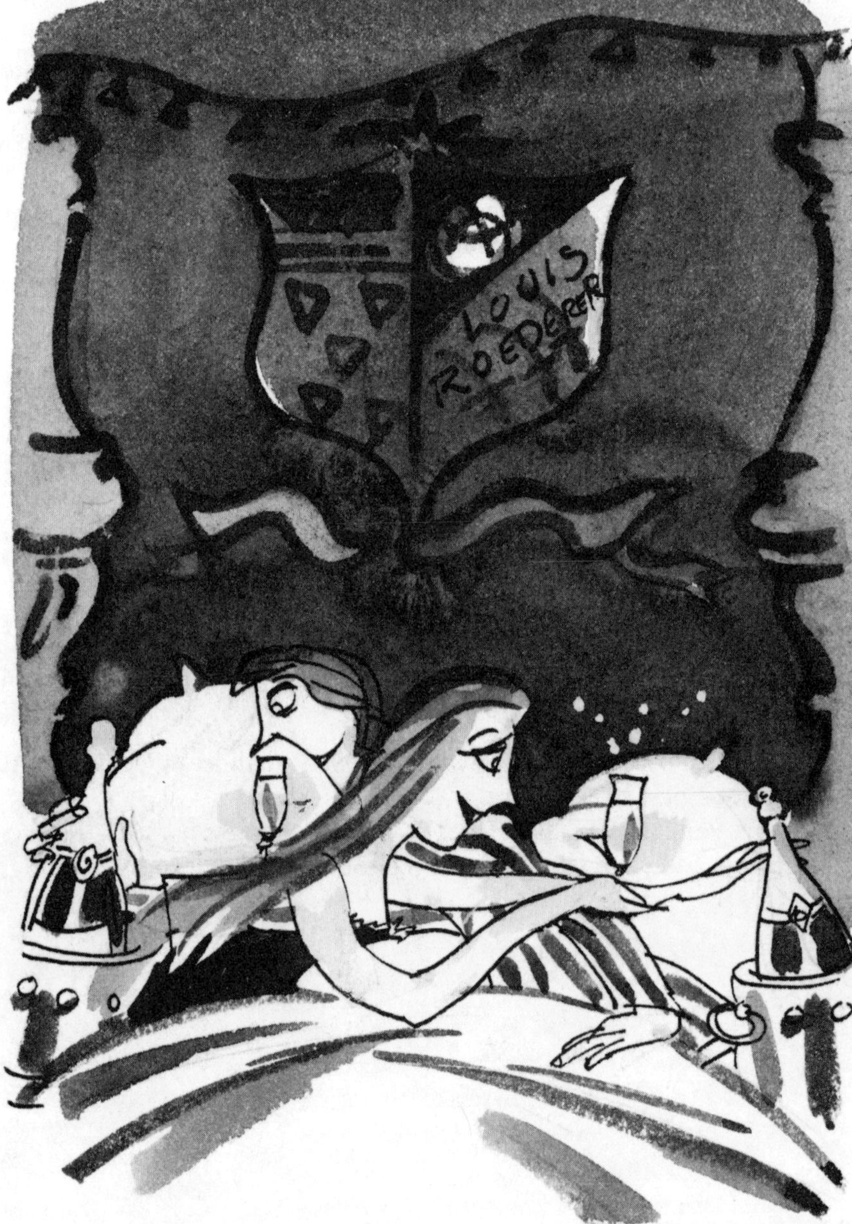

a scene from Dynasty

Envoi

You have lost what you set out to lose, the pounds (in weight & sterling) have been shed and the stomach muscles tightened. It's a fine figure which now smiles out at you from a full-length mirror. A reward is due and what better than the sybaratic indulgence of breakfast in bed, mid-morning.

Dress for the occasion in satin pyjamas or a negligee, refresh the pulse points with Guerlain's Dry Imperial, the Cologne that Napolean III bathed with before going into battle.

As you will be sharing this event, hopefully with an adoring companion, the occasion calls for a little 'extra something', a jar of Beluga caviar sunk in a silver bowl filled with crushed ice, the moist blue-black eggs to be tantalizingly nibbled on delicate triangles of toast. Hot brioches would be succulent if their centres had been removed and replaced with warm foie gras. These little delicacies should be accompanied by a bottle of Louis Roederer, or even better, two bottles of Louis Roederer's Cristal, one on either side of the bed. Reaching across your partner to get the Champagne out of the ice bucket is good exercise for the arm, chest and torso.

Cristal, made from the finest grapes, was originally created for Tsar Alexander II of Russia who like his Champagne bottles to be made out of pure cyrstal. The Champagne was named after the Tsar's choice of bottle.

The illustration might remind you of a scene from *Dynasty*, if it does, you're right, Alexis and Dex always have Champagne both sides of the bed just in case they get thirsty discussing oil leases.

This book has not only introduced you to the Champagne Diet but also to the Champagne Philosophy of Life. As a man of great style, but slender means, said with commendable dignity, as he savoured a glass of particularly elegant Henriot Cuvée Baccarat: 'He who drinks beer, thinks beer and, I am happy to say, I have never let a drop pass my lips.'